4TH
EDITION

NETTER'S
ATLAS of ANATOMY for
SPEECH, SWALLOWING,
and HEARING

4TH
EDITION

NETTER'S ATLAS of ANATOMY for SPEECH, SWALLOWING, and HEARING

David H. McFarland

Professor
School of Speech Language Pathology and Audiology
Faculty of Medicine
University of Montreal;
Adjunct Professor
School of Communication Sciences and Disorders
Faculty of Medicine
McGill University
Montreal, Quebec, Canada

ELSEVIER

Elsevier
1600 John F. Kennedy Blvd.
Ste 1800
Philadelphia, PA 19103-2899

NETTER'S ATLAS OF ANATOMY FOR SPEECH, SWALLOWING,
AND HEARING, FOURTH EDITION

ISBN: 978-0-323830348

Notice

Practitioners and researchers must always rely on their own experience and knowledge in evaluating and
using any information, methods, compounds or experiments described herein. Because of rapid advances in
the medical sciences, in particular, independent verification of diagnoses and drug dosages should be made.
To the fullest extent of the law, no responsibility is assumed by Elsevier, authors, editors or contributors for
any injury and/or damage to persons or property as a matter of products liability, negligence or otherwise, or
from any use or operation of any methods, products, instructions, or ideas contained in the material herein.

Publisher: Elyse W. O'Grady
Director, Content Development: Rebecca Gruliow
Publishing Service Manager: Shereen Jameel
Senior Project Manager: Beula Christopher
Design Direction: Patrick C. Ferguson

Printed in India
Last digit is the print number: 9 8 7 6 5 4 3 2

PREFACE

Speech, swallowing, hearing, and balance are human behaviors that are vital to everyday life. Diagnosing and treating their disordered function requires a thorough understanding of the many body systems involved.

The purpose of this atlas is to provide readers with a comprehensive reference for the essential aspects of speech, swallowing, hearing, and vestibular anatomy. Key physiological and nervous system processes, which cannot be dissociated from anatomy, have also been summarized to deliver a more complete picture of these functions. This fourth edition was an opportunity to greatly expand content and create and include five more key anatomical illustrations.

■ AUDIENCE

This atlas is for anyone interested in the body systems involved in speech, swallowing, hearing, and balance, either for understanding normal processes or as a basis for clinical practice. It is specifically tailored for instructors and students in both undergraduate and graduate programs, in addition for researchers and clinicians in the fields of speech-language pathology, audiology, and related medical disciplines. My sincere ambition for this book is that it will serve as a useful learning tool for students and be a faithful reference for practitioners and researchers. I also hope that it will become a functional guide for clinicians who work with disorders of speech, swallowing, and hearing and used to educate patients suffering from these problems. Perhaps one day it may even become a platform for shared communication among the diverse professionals encountering the challenges of these complex disorders.

■ CONCEPT AND IMPORTANCE TO THE PROFESSION

The inaugural edition of this atlas was the first time that the medical illustrations of Frank Netter had been gathered into a volume dedicated to speech, swallowing, and hearing. These seminal illustrations were chosen in part because they are used extensively in other disciplines and thereby represent a common base of study and clinical reference for students, instructors, and professionals in these fields. The images also have garnered the favor of scholars and clinicians because they provide just the right level of detail and clearly convey the relationship among key anatomical structures. We have been fortunate in this fourth edition to be able to supplement and update some of the Netter illustrations and to create new images highlighting key aspects of structure and function.

■ ORGANIZATION

For the physiological component of the book, I adopted a targeted approach to provide essential information that is useful and appropriate for clinical practice. Clear parallels are made between the structure being referenced on the left page and the accompanying illustration on the right. Each section concludes with summary tables featuring key muscles or cranial nerves. Core physiological concepts were reviewed and greatly expanded upon in this fourth edition.

Ease of use was one of my main organizational objectives. Because education is one of the primary purposes of this work, the content reflects the way the anatomy and physiology of speech and swallowing are traditionally taught. It begins with a basic introduction to anatomy and moves on to a more detailed discussion of the three key systems involved in speech, voice, and swallowing—the respiratory, laryngeal-phonatory, and oropharyngeal-articulatory systems. It concludes by covering fundamental hearing, vestibular, and neurological systems.

■ DISTINCTIVE FEATURES

- *Full-Color Presentation:* This is the first and only atlas of anatomy specific to speech, swallowing, and hearing to include full-color Netter images, providing maximum detail and accuracy for students and clinicians.
- *Stellar Art Program:* The remarkable, time-honored, and detailed images of renowned illustrator Dr. Frank Netter take center stage in this atlas. Dr. Netter's artwork has been used for years to teach leading health care professionals and researchers. Images are presented from various orientations and levels of detail to ensure that readers gain the foundation they need to work with patients who have disorders of speech, swallowing, and hearing.
- *Atlas Format:* Information on targeted anatomical and related physiological mechanisms is found on the left page, with a corresponding image detailing the related anatomy on the right page. This "read-it, see-it" approach appeals to a wide variety of learning styles and makes it ideal for clinical reference.
- *Instruction-Based Organization:* The organization of the sections follows a logical order that is consistent with the way this content is taught in educational programs—an overview of anatomy followed by successive sections detailing the anatomy and related physiology of the respiratory, laryngeal-phonatory, oropharyngeal-articulatory, auditory and vestibulatory, and nervous systems—making it an ideal complement to any related courses.
- *Appropriate Depth of Coverage:* The text—often presented in a bulleted-list style for easy reference and comprehension—presents readers with the essential, need-to-know information relevant to speech, swallowing, and hearing and vestibular mechanisms. This unique and targeted approach provides just the right level of depth and detail to give the artwork proper context.
- *Summary Muscular Tables:* The chapters on the respiratory, laryngeal-phonatory, and oropharyngeal-articulatory systems conclude with tables detailing the relevant musculature of that body system, which include the origin, insertion, innervation, and action of each. The chapter on the nervous system concludes with a table detailing the cranial nerves most significant for speech, mastication/swallowing, and hearing/balance. These tables present vital information in a quick, easy, and consistent format ideal for study or quick reference.

■ ANCILLARIES

A companion Evolve website (http://evolve.elsevier.com/McFarland/Netter) has been developed to accompany this book with tools to enhance teaching for instructors and learning for students.

■ INSTRUCTOR RESOURCES

- *Test Bank:* Approximately 275 objective-style questions—multiple-choice, true/false, fill-in-the-blank, and matching—with accompanying rationales for correct answers and page-number or page-range references for remediation.

■ STUDENT RESOURCES

- *Self-Test Questions:* Approximately 150 objective-style questions—multiple-choice, true/false, fill-in-the-blank, and matching—are available for examination preparation and accompanied by instant feedback and remediation assistance.
- *Labeling Exercises:* Many of the book's illustrations have been turned into interactive exercises as a practice tool to help students master the relevant anatomy.

David H. McFarland

ACKNOWLEDGEMENTS

They say a picture is worth a thousand words. I decided to add words anyway to these classic anatomical images after my students told me that a tool like this would be invaluable to them in their training as speech-language pathologists.

It is hard to imagine that what started out as a simple teaching tool would now be a book in its fourth edition with versions in French, Spanish, Portuguese, Greek, and Chinese. This has been a remarkable journey and one that would not have been possible without the motivation of students past and present and of exceptional colleagues who have reviewed key sections of the book for accuracy, completeness, and clinical relevance.

This fourth edition includes additional key information on the auditory system, most notably the anatomy of the vestibular system. The oropharyngeal-articulatory system has been revised and expanded, and an overview of the procedures that make it possible to visualize vocal tract structures has been added. The chapter on the nervous system was increased to provide important additional details on motor pathways, spinal nerves, cerebral circulation, and the cortical innervation of cranial and spinal nerves. Five key medical illustrations were added, one illustrating the anatomy of the vestibular system; one to illustrate the sensory innervation of the larynx, pharynx, and the oral and nasal cavities; one to show the extensive anatomical overlap of the physiological systems involved in speech and swallowing; and one to illustrate the zone of apposition between the diaphragm and rib cage. A final addition is a static radiographic image of the head and neck to orient readers to those anatomical structures typically visualized in videofluoroscopic examinations of swallowing.

In addition to all of the persons who have contributed to past editions, I would like to thank Kate Davidson, Dr. Bonnie Martin-Harris, Dr. William Pearson, and Daniel Piché for the assistance in the creation of the illustration of the static radiographic image of the head and neck.

A very special thank you to Simone Poulin and Annie Joëlle Fortin for the invaluable support they gave to ensure that this fourth edition was of the highest quality.

Finally, I would like to thank my colleagues at Elsevier, as well as the students, clinicians, and faculty around the world who use this reference book for educational purposes or to support their clinical work with people with speech, voice, language, and swallowing disorders. I am very grateful for the trust you place in my book. It is an honor to guide you through the wonderful world of clinical speech-language pathology anatomy and physiology.

TABLE OF CONTENTS

INTRODUCTION

Speech differs from many other skilled human movements in that the goal is not to move the body or interact with an object, but to communicate. It has been estimated that we may produce up to 15 speech sounds per second, which may require the activity of approximately 100 muscles distributed across the different physiological systems involved in speech production, including the respiratory, laryngeal, and oral-articulatory systems. The use of these different systems makes speech production one of the most complex of all human skilled movements. The underlying neural control processes are similarly complex and involve several hierarchically organized cortical and subcortical structures interacting with sensory feedback from peripheral speech structures. As illustrated in Figure 1 [p. 2], swallowing uses many, if not all, of the same anatomical structures (and neural control processes) that are involved in speech production, but for different purposes. For example, the vocal folds, crucial for sound production for speech, are key elements in protecting the airway during swallowing. The oral articulators that shape the sound produced by the vibrating folds are used in the preparation and transportation of foods and liquids for swallowing. The pharynx, part of the vocal tract, moves the swallowed bolus toward the esophagus and stomach. Given this high degree of anatomical overlap, it is not surprising that disease or damage affecting speech may also affect swallowing.

The goal of this book is to summarize our current understanding of the anatomical basis of normal speech, voice, and swallowing function and to provide a platform for the diagnosis and treatment of disorders of these vital behaviors. This is combined with an introduction to hearing and vestibular functional anatomy. Physiology is briefly summarized because structure and function are intimately related and are only artificially separated in this book to simplify learning.

This book is organized around the pioneering medical illustrations of Frank M. Netter. Anatomical descriptions are presented with specific reference to these classic illustrations, and the relevant structures are highlighted. Understanding anatomy requires a visual representation of structure from various orientations, and Netter's figures provide this thorough perspective. Summary tables of muscle origin, insertion, innervation, and function are provided throughout. Figures from other talented illustrators have been added throughout the different editions of this book to highlight key structure and function. In this edition, we have added our original figures to orient the learner to understanding the anatomical structures observable in a videofluoroscopic assessment of swallowing.

We begin with an overview of anatomical classification systems, a summary of anatomical nomenclature, a list of the terms used to describe direction and movement, and a description of the different types of anatomical tissues. We continue with descriptions of the respiratory, laryngeal, and oropharyngeal structures and end with hearing anatomy and key neurological systems involved in the control and coordination of speech and swallowing movements.

The study of anatomy is one of the oldest medical sciences, and its origins can be traced back to at least the early Greeks. You are embarking on this grand and noble tradition in the study of human anatomical principles.

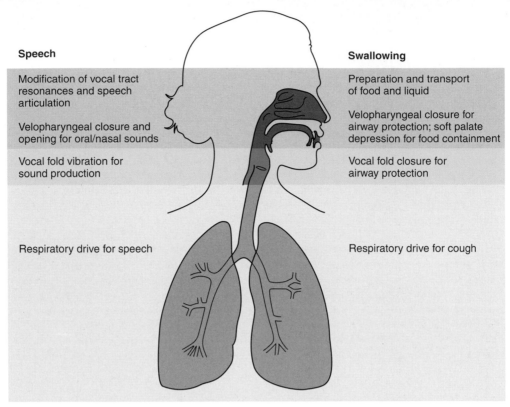

Speech

Modification of vocal tract resonances and speech articulation

Velopharyngeal closure and opening for oral/nasal sounds

Vocal fold vibration for sound production

Respiratory drive for speech

Swallowing

Preparation and transport of food and liquid

Velopharyngeal closure for airway protection; soft palate depression for food containment

Vocal fold closure for airway protection

Respiratory drive for cough

Figure 1 Shared anatomical structures involved in speech and swallowing.

■ ANATOMY

There are many ways of classifying and consequently studying anatomy. Some of these are described in the next sections. This book uses many of these methods to cover the following aspects of anatomy in relation to speech, swallowing, and hearing:

- The normal structure of organs and systems
- The topographical or anatomical relationships between structures
- The function of anatomical structures
- The development of anatomical structures and systems
- The neurological aspects of a structure's normal function
- Certain clinical aspects of disordered function

Systemic Anatomy

Systemic anatomy classifies the body by biological systems and subsystems. The major systems include the integumentary system, the skeletal system, the muscular system, the articular system, the nervous system, the circulatory system, the respiratory system, the digestive system, the urinary system, the reproductive system, and the endocrine system.

Regional Anatomy

Regional anatomy emphasizes the different regions or divisions of the body and the relationship between the anatomical structures of those divisions. The typical regions are as follows:

- Head and neck
- Back
- Thorax
- Abdomen
- Pelvis and perineum
- Upper limb
- Lower limb

Developmental Anatomy

Developmental anatomy concerns the prenatal and postnatal development of anatomical structures.

Functional Anatomy

Functional anatomy classifies the relationship between a structure and its function, combining anatomy and physiology.

Clinical Anatomy

Clinical anatomy emphasizes the relationship between anatomy and medical or other clinical practice.

■ NOMENCLATURE

Before beginning to discuss the human body, it is important to know the terms most frequently used by anatomists to describe a structure and its location. These terms greatly facilitate the understanding and study of anatomy.

Anatomical Position (Figure 2)

All structures are described in relationship to a standard position, which is called the *anatomical position.* In *humans,* the anatomical position is standing, facing the observer, arms along the body, palms turned forward, legs together or slightly separated, and feet straight ahead.

Because most nonhuman animals are on all fours, their anatomical position and terms of direction are different from those of humans. This should be kept in mind when comparing nonhuman with human anatomy.

■ PLANES AND SECTIONS

Anatomical planes divide the body into different sections and are used to describe structures and anatomical movements. To visualize these different planes, we will ask you to imagine a sheet of paper that "cuts" the body into different sections. Following is a description of the three main anatomical reference planes (see Figure 2).

Sagittal

The sagittal plane is a longitudinal plane that is parallel to the sagittal suture of the skull. To visualize this plane, imagine the sheet of paper aligned vertically between your eyes. All sagittal planes are parallel to this sheet. The *median* or *midsagittal* plane is the sagittal plane that divides the body into two equal left and right halves. All other sagittal planes or sections are termed *parasagittal,* or just *sagittal.*

Frontal or Coronal

The frontal, or coronal, plane is a longitudinal plane that crosses the sagittal plane at a right angle. To visualize this plane, imagine holding the sheet of paper directly in front of you and parallel to the coronal or frontal suture of the cranium. All frontal planes will be parallel to this sheet. Coronal planes divide the body front to back (anteriorly to posteriorly). The terms *midfrontal* or *midcoronal* are sometimes used to designate the plane that divides the body into equal anterior and posterior halves.

Transverse or Horizontal

The transverse, or horizontal, plane divides the body or structure into superior/inferior portions. To visualize this plane, imagine the sheet of paper placed horizontally in front of your face that divides your head into upper and lower halves. All transverse planes are parallel to this sheet. The term *midtransverse* is used to designate the plane dividing the body into two equal superior and inferior halves.

NOTE: An oblique plane is oriented obliquely between one of the planes described here.

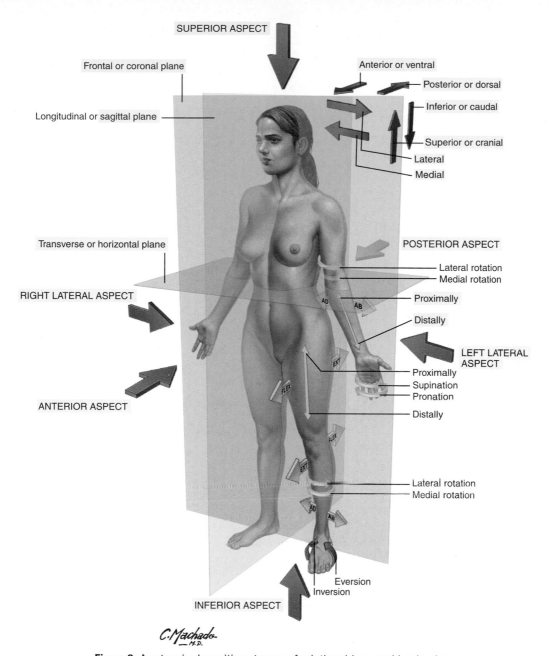

SUPERIOR ASPECT

Frontal or coronal plane

Anterior or ventral

Posterior or dorsal

Longitudinal or sagittal plane

Inferior or caudal

Superior or cranial

Lateral

Medial

Transverse or horizontal plane

POSTERIOR ASPECT

Lateral rotation
Medial rotation

RIGHT LATERAL ASPECT

Proximally

Distally

AD   AB

LEFT LATERAL
ASPECT

EXT

Proximally
Supination
Pronation

FLEX

Distally

ANTERIOR ASPECT

FLEX

EXT

Lateral rotation
Medial rotation

AD   AB

Eversion
Inversion

INFERIOR ASPECT

C. Machado
—M.D.

Figure 2 Anatomical position, terms of relationships, and body planes.

NOTE: Labels of certain figures are highlighted in yellow to emphasize the related elements in the corresponding text.

■ ANATOMICAL TERMS

Directional terms are used to locate anatomical structures and to explain the spatial relationship between structures relative to the anatomical position. They are presented in contrasting pairs (see Figure 2 [p. 5] – refer to the purple and blue arrows).

Superior and Inferior

- Superior (rostral, cranial) is toward the upper portion or located above a structure of the body.
- Inferior (caudal) is toward the lower portion or below a structure of the body.

Anterior and Posterior

- Anterior (ventral) is toward the front or in front of a structure of the body.
- Posterior (dorsal) is toward the back or behind a structure of the body.

Medial, Lateral, and Median

- Medial is toward the midline, or central axis, of the body.
- Lateral is away from the central axis, or midline, of the body.
- Median is on the central sagittal plane.

Proximal and Distal

- Proximal is toward the origin of a structure of the body.
- Distal is away from the origin of a structure of the body. Proximal and distal are often used to describe the limbs.

External, Internal, and Intermediate

- External (superficial) is toward the surface of a structure of the body.
- Internal (deep) is away from the surface of a structure of the body.
- Intermediate (middle) is between internal and external.

   These terms are often used to describe anatomical relationships between structures, such as one structure being deep to or superficial to another.

Parietal and Visceral (see Figure 6 [p. 11])

- Parietal is the outer layer or covering of a body cavity.
- Visceral is the inner layer of a cavity wrapped around body organs.

Prone and Supine

- Prone is the anatomical position of the body with the face and ventral surface of the body facing down.
- Supine is the anatomical position of the body with the face and ventral surface of the body facing up.

Ipsilateral, Contralateral, and Bilateral

- Ipsilateral refers to the same side of the body.
- Contralateral refers to the opposite side of the body.
- Bilateral refers to both sides of the body.

   Note that the terms ipsilateral, contralateral, and bilateral are commonly used in reference to the innervation of a structure. Innervation is the supply or distribution of motor and/or sensory nerves to or from an organ, muscle, or gland.

■ VIEWS, ASPECTS, AND SURFACES

Anatomy requires the visualization of structures from different perspectives. The terms *view, aspect,* and *surface* are used to describe these orientations. A view describes how we are oriented to observe the body or a structure (see Figure 2 [p. 5] – refer to the red arrows):

- A superior view is when the observer is positioned above a structure, whereas an inferior view is when the observer is positioned below a structure (see Figure 3 [p. 8]).
- An anterior view is when the observer is positioned in the front of a structure, whereas a posterior view is when the observer is positioned behind a structure (see Figures 4 [p. 9] and 6 [p. 11]).
- A lateral view is when the observer is positioned farther from the median plane of the body (see "Sagittal," p. 4), whereas a medial view is when the observer is positioned directly on the median plane (see Figures 4 [p. 9] and 5 [p. 10]).

Surface refers to the outside/uppermost layers of an anatomical structure (e.g., see the anterior surface of the lungs in Figure 6 [p. 11]). Aspect refers to that part of an anatomical structure viewed from a particular direction (see the lateral aspect of the skull in a lateral view, as shown in Figure 5 [p. 10]).

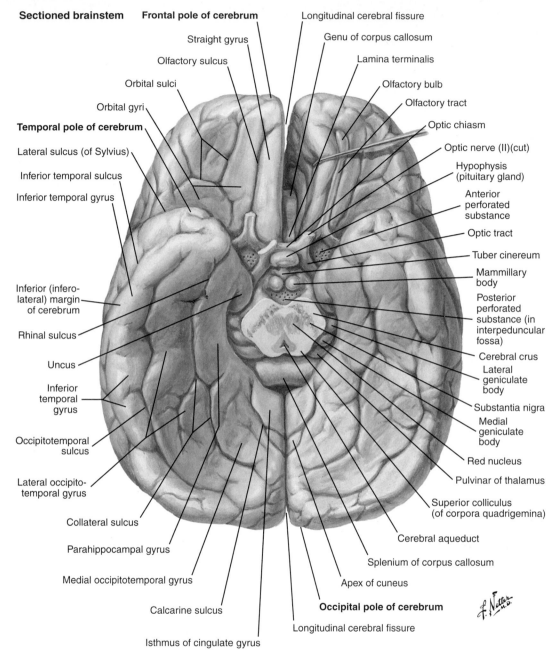

Sectioned brainstem   **Frontal pole of cerebrum**   Longitudinal cerebral fissure

Straight gyrus   Genu of corpus callosum

Olfactory sulcus   Lamina terminalis

Orbital sulci   Olfactory bulb

Orbital gyri   Olfactory tract

Temporal pole of cerebrum   Optic chiasm

Lateral sulcus (of Sylvius)   Optic nerve (II)(cut)

Inferior temporal sulcus   Hypophysis (pituitary gland)

Inferior temporal gyrus   Anterior perforated substance

Optic tract

Tuber cinereum

Mammillary body

Inferior (inferolateral) margin of cerebrum   Posterior perforated substance (in interpeduncular fossa)

Rhinal sulcus   Cerebral crus

Uncus   Lateral geniculate body

Inferior temporal gyrus   Substantia nigra

Medial geniculate body

Occipitotemporal sulcus   Red nucleus

Lateral occipito-temporal gyrus   Pulvinar of thalamus

Superior colliculus (of corpora quadrigemina)

Collateral sulcus   Cerebral aqueduct

Parahippocampal gyrus   Splenium of corpus callosum

Medial occipitotemporal gyrus   Apex of cuneus

Calcarine sulcus   **Occipital pole of cerebrum**

Longitudinal cerebral fissure

Isthmus of cingulate gyrus

Figure 3 Inferior view of the cerebrum.

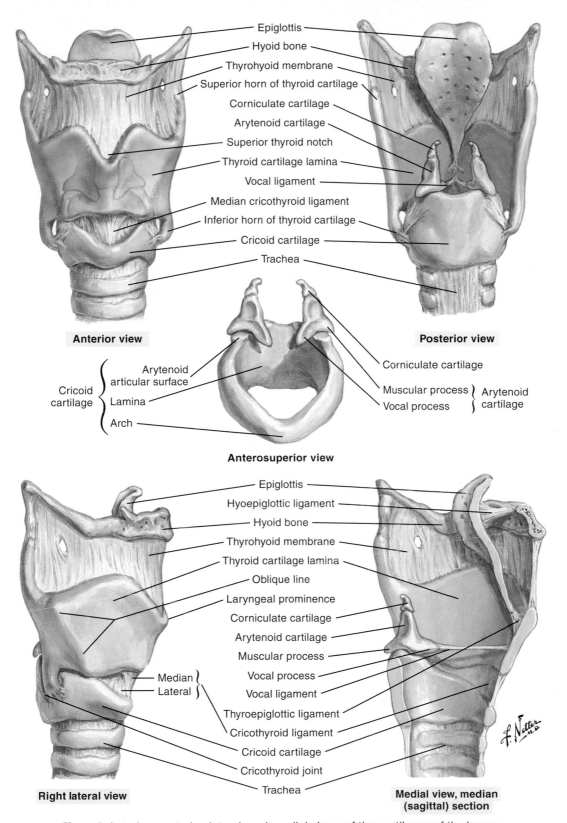

Epiglottis
Hyoid bone
Thyrohyoid membrane
Superior horn of thyroid cartilage
Corniculate cartilage
Arytenoid cartilage
Superior thyroid notch
Thyroid cartilage lamina
Vocal ligament
Median cricothyroid ligament
Inferior horn of thyroid cartilage
Cricoid cartilage
Trachea

Anterior view

Posterior view

Cricoid cartilage
Arytenoid articular surface
Lamina
Arch

Corniculate cartilage
Muscular process
Vocal process
Arytenoid cartilage

Anterosuperior view

Epiglottis
Hyoepiglottic ligament
Hyoid bone
Thyrohyoid membrane
Thyroid cartilage lamina
Oblique line
Laryngeal prominence
Corniculate cartilage
Arytenoid cartilage
Muscular process
Vocal process
Vocal ligament
Thyroepiglottic ligament
Cricothyroid ligament
Cricoid cartilage
Cricothyroid joint
Trachea

Median
Lateral

Right lateral view

Medial view, median (sagittal) section

Figure 4 Anterior, posterior, lateral, and medial views of the cartilages of the larynx.

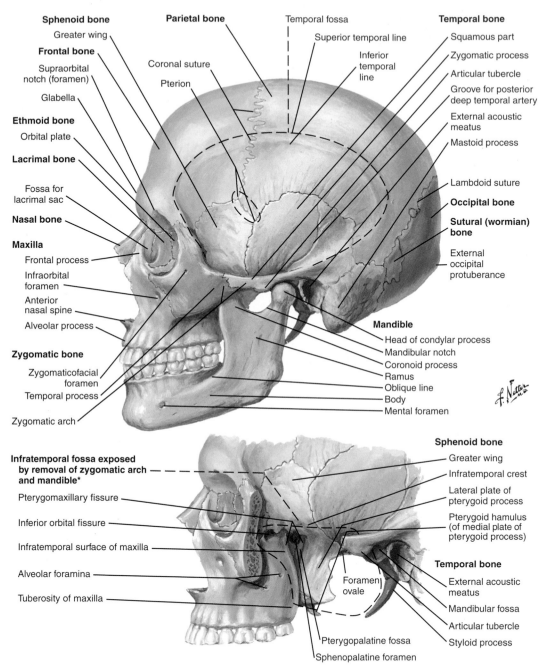

Sphenoid bone
Greater wing
Frontal bone
Supraorbital notch (foramen)
Glabella
Ethmoid bone
Orbital plate
Lacrimal bone
Fossa for lacrimal sac
Nasal bone
Maxilla
Frontal process
Infraorbital foramen
Anterior nasal spine
Alveolar process
Zygomatic bone
Zygomaticofacial foramen
Temporal process
Zygomatic arch

Parietal bone
Coronal suture
Pterion

Temporal fossa
Superior temporal line
Inferior temporal line

Temporal bone
Squamous part
Zygomatic process
Articular tubercle
Groove for posterior deep temporal artery
External acoustic meatus
Mastoid process
Lambdoid suture
Occipital bone
Sutural (wormian) bone
External occipital protuberance

Mandible
Head of condylar process
Mandibular notch
Coronoid process
Ramus
Oblique line
Body
Mental foramen

Infratemporal fossa exposed by removal of zygomatic arch and mandible*
Pterygomaxillary fissure
Inferior orbital fissure
Infratemporal surface of maxilla
Alveolar foramina
Tuberosity of maxilla

Sphenoid bone
Greater wing
Infratemporal crest
Lateral plate of pterygoid process
Pterygoid hamulus (of medial plate of pterygoid process)
Temporal bone
External acoustic meatus
Mandibular fossa
Articular tubercle
Styloid process

Foramen ovale
Pterygopalatine fossa
Sphenopalatine foramen

*Superficially, mastoid process forms posterior boundary.

Figure 5 Lateral view of the skull.

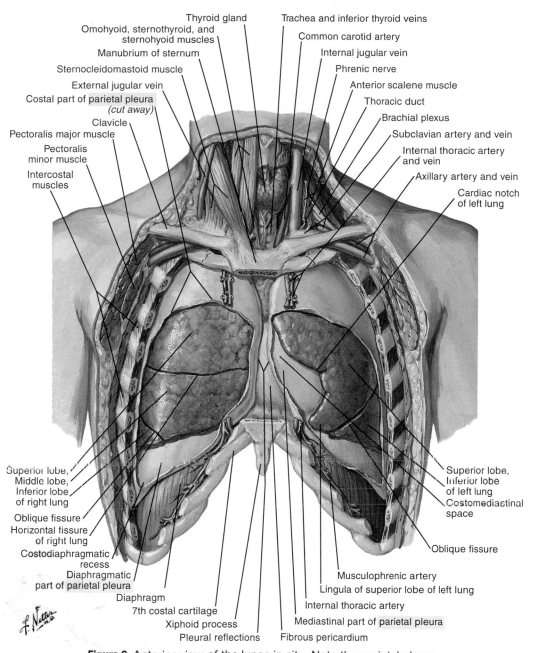

Thyroid gland

Trachea and inferior thyroid veins

Omohyoid, sternothyroid, and sternohyoid muscles

Common carotid artery

Manubrium of sternum

Internal jugular vein

Sternocleidomastoid muscle

Phrenic nerve

External jugular vein

Anterior scalene muscle

Costal part of parietal pleura *(cut away)*

Thoracic duct

Clavicle

Brachial plexus

Pectoralis major muscle

Subclavian artery and vein

Pectoralis minor muscle

Internal thoracic artery and vein

Intercostal muscles

Axillary artery and vein

Cardiac notch of left lung

Superior lobe, Middle lobe, Inferior lobe of right lung

Superior lobe, Inferior lobe of left lung

Oblique fissure

Costomediastinal space

Horizontal fissure of right lung

Costodiaphragmatic recess

Diaphragmatic part of parietal pleura

Oblique fissure

Diaphragm

Musculophrenic artery

7th costal cartilage

Lingula of superior lobe of left lung

Xiphoid process

Internal thoracic artery

Pleural reflections

Fibrous pericardium

Mediastinal part of parietal pleura

Figure 6 Anterior view of the lungs in situ. Note the parietal pleura.

■ ANATOMICAL MOVEMENT

As with terms of direction, anatomical movements are usually described in contrasting pairs. Each pair is detailed in the following sections (see Figure 2 [p. 5]).

Flexion and Extension

- Flexion is the movement around a joint that brings two adjacent bones or body segments closer together, reducing the angle of articulation.
- Extension is the movement around a joint that brings two adjacent bones or body segments farther apart, increasing the angle of articulation.

Abduction and Adduction

- Abduction is the movement of a structure away from the midline.
- Adduction is the movement of a structure toward the midline.

Elevation and Depression

- Elevation is the upward movement of a structure.
- Depression is the downward movement of a structure.

Protrusion and Retrusion

- Protrusion (protraction) is the forward movement of a structure.
- Retrusion (retraction) is the backward movement of a structure.

Supination and Pronation

Supination and pronation refer to rotational movements of certain structures such as the arm and hand:

- Supination refers to the rotation of the arm and hand so that the palm is facing anteriorly (with arm straight) or upward (with arm bent).
- Pronation refers to the rotation of the arm and hand so that the palm is facing posteriorly (with arm straight) or downward (with arm bent).

■ VOCABULARY SPECIFIC TO ANATOMY

Many structures are named according to either their anatomical location on the body (e.g., external intercostal muscles, supraglottic, and so on) or their function (e.g., levator scapulae muscle, depressor anguli oris muscle, and so on). In addition to their anatomical name, other structures have names originating from mythology (e.g., Achilles tendon) or from the first person who associated the structure with a disease or a malformation or the first person who described the structure (e.g., circle of Willis).

Names of muscles and ligaments may also correspond to their points of attachment, as follows:

- Origin corresponds to the point of attachment of a muscle that remains relatively fixed during muscular contraction.
- Insertion corresponds to the more mobile point of attachment.

In general, the origin is named first and the insertion second. Sometimes, origin and insertion can be interchanged (insertion first and origin second) if both are considered of equal mobility. Muscle names may also provide information about the form of the muscle, such as the number of bellies or portions of the muscle (e.g., *di*gastric, or two bellies), its overall shape or location (e.g., *external* intercostals), or its action (e.g., *tensor* veli palatini).

■ PRIMARY TISSUES

Tissues are groups of cells with similar structure that perform a common function. The four primary tissue groups are as follows:

1. Epithelial
2. Connective
3. Muscular
4. Nervous

Epithelial Tissue (Epithelium, Epithelia)

Epithelia cover surfaces of the body and the body cavities of different systems (respiratory, digestive, cardiac, and vascular systems). This group of tissue performs the following functions:

- Protection
- Absorption and filtration
- Excretion and secretion
- Sensation

Connective Tissue

Connective tissue is a key component (with muscles and the skeleton) of the musculoskeletal system. It is widespread in the human body, and its principal functions are as follows:

- Fixation and support
- Protection
- Energy reserve
- Transportation of fluids and other substances

   Connective tissue can be solid, liquid, or gelatinous and can be classified in several different ways. Connective tissues are generally divided into two main categories: (1) connective tissues proper and (2) specialized connective tissues.

Connective Tissues Proper

This type of connective tissue includes different subcategories depending on the type, amount and arrangement of the cells, fibers, and extracellular matrix that compose them. The following classification is presented, but there are several other ways to group the different subcategories. It should also be noted that types of tissue are more of a continuum than discrete entities.

Loose

- **Areolar** connective tissue is a supple and gelatinous tissue formed of collagen and elastin fibers that surrounds and forms a cushion for organs and other body structures.
- **Adipose** connective tissue is composed of adipose cells and stores fat, protects and supports certain organs, and acts as an insulator.
- **Reticular** connective tissue is similar to areolar tissue and is composed only of reticular fibers. It forms the stroma, which has a supporting function in lymphoid and hematopoietic organs (e.g., lymph nodes and bone marrow).

Dense

- **Dense regular** connective tissue is composed primarily of collagen fibers and some elastic fibers that follow a parallel orientation. It interconnects and supports body structures. Collagen fibers are quite stiff relative to elastic fibers and take longer to recover from deformation (like stretch). Tendons, ligaments, fascia, and aponeuroses are composed of dense regular connective tissue.
- **Dense irregular** connective tissue is principally composed of collagen fibers with no specific orientation and few elastic fibers. Its function is to reinforce and protect. Dense irregular connective tissue is found in the deep fascia of the body, the joint capsules, and the dermis (skin).
- **Elastic** connective tissue has a high concentration of elastic fibers (elastin and others), which confer flexibility and resistance. Such tissues are found in the bronchial tree and larynx, including the vocal ligament of the vocal folds.

Specialized Connective Tissues

The following types of connective tissue are categorized separately, as their structure and function are highly specialized.

Cartilage

- **Hyaline** cartilage is the most common cartilage. It contains collagen fibers and provides strength and flexibility. Some examples are costal, nasal, tracheal, and most laryngeal cartilages.
- **Elastic** cartilage is similar to hyaline cartilage but contains more elastic fibers and is thus more flexible. Some examples are the external ear, pharyngotympanic tube, epiglottis, and cuneiform and corniculate cartilages.
- **Fibrocartilage** is composed of dense collagen fibers and provides strength and shock absorption. Examples are the intervertebral discs and pubic symphysis.

More detail is provided on the following types of connective tissues that appear frequently in the atlas:

- **Membranes** are layers of epithelial and/or connective tissue that cover and protect body cavities and other surfaces. There are four types of membranes: mucous, serous, synovial, and cutaneous.
- **Tendons** are strong bands of dense regular connective tissue that connect skeletal muscle to bone. Tendons are flexible but resist extension (stretch). They are supplied with important sensory nerve endings: the Golgi tendon organs.
- **Aponeuroses** are broad tendinous-like sheets that cover muscle or are the points of origin or insertion of skeletal muscle.
- **Ligaments** are strong bands of dense regular connective tissue that connect bone to bone, cartilage to cartilage, and cartilage to bone. Ligaments are slightly elastic ("stretchy") and lengthen under tension.
- **Fascia** is connective tissue that covers and groups anatomical structures (muscles and organs) and also serves as a point of attachment of some muscles.

Osseous Tissue

Osseous tissue is hard and rigid tissue that is composed of collagen fibers and minerals. Bones produce red and white blood cells, store minerals, support the body, protect vital organs, and provide skeletal support for movement. They also serve a sound transmission role in bone-conducted hearing.

Blood

Although a fluid, blood is classified as a specialized connective tissue. It is composed of red blood cells, white blood cells, and platelets suspended in plasma. It transports respiratory gases, nutrients, and other substances crucial for normal body functions.

Muscular Tissue

- **Skeletal** muscles are composed of striated muscle fibers and are involved in the production of movements.
- **Cardiac** muscles are composed of striated cells and have involuntary control of the heart.
- **Smooth** muscles are composed of nonstriated cells and are involved in the involuntary control of body organs.

Nervous Tissue

The nervous system is composed of the following types of nervous tissue:
- Neurons are specialized cells that conduct nerve impulses.
- Glial cells are nonconducting cells that support, insulate, and protect neurons.

■ TERMS RELATIVE TO BONES

Terms relative to bones are classified into the following categories:
1. Depressions
2. Elevations

Depressions

- A fissure is a cleft.
- A foramen is a natural opening (Figures 7 and 8 [p. 18]).
- A fossa is a depression (see Figure 8 [p. 18]).
- A groove is a furrow (see Figure 8 [p. 18]).
- A meatus is a passageway (see Figures 8 [p. 18] and 9 [p. 19]).
- A sinus is a cavity (see Figure 9 [p. 19]).

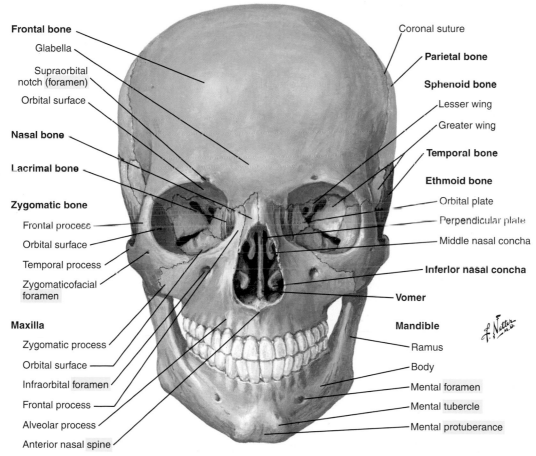

Figure 7 Anterior view of the skull, showing examples of the foramen, tubercle, spine, and protuberance.

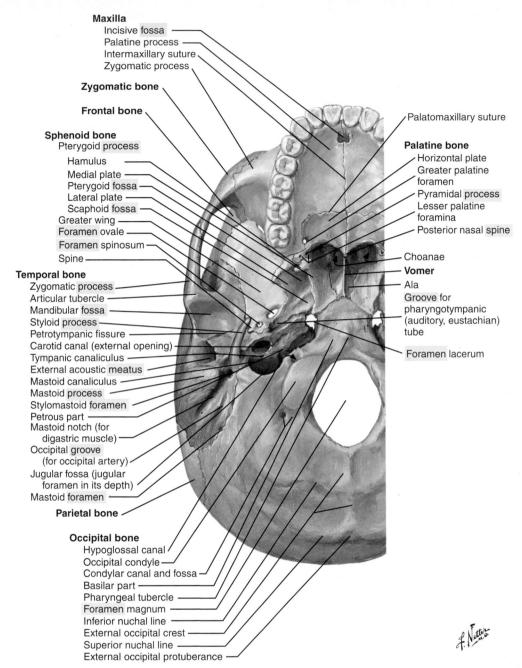

Maxilla
Incisive fossa
Palatine process
Intermaxillary suture
Zygomatic process

Zygomatic bone

Frontal bone

Sphenoid bone
Pterygoid process
Hamulus
Medial plate
Pterygoid fossa
Lateral plate
Scaphoid fossa
Greater wing
Foramen ovale
Foramen spinosum
Spine

Temporal bone
Zygomatic process
Articular tubercle
Mandibular fossa
Styloid process
Petrotympanic fissure
Carotid canal (external opening)
Tympanic canaliculus
External acoustic meatus
Mastoid canaliculus
Mastoid process
Stylomastoid foramen
Petrous part
Mastoid notch (for
digastric muscle)
Occipital groove
(for occipital artery)
Jugular fossa (jugular
foramen in its depth)
Mastoid foramen

Parietal bone

Occipital bone
Hypoglossal canal
Occipital condyle
Condylar canal and fossa
Basilar part
Pharyngeal tubercle
Foramen magnum
Inferior nuchal line
External occipital crest
Superior nuchal line
External occipital protuberance

Palatomaxillary suture

Palatine bone
Horizontal plate
Greater palatine
foramen
Pyramidal process
Lesser palatine
foramina
Posterior nasal spine

Choanae
Vomer
Ala
Groove for
pharyngotympanic
(auditory, eustachian)
tube

Foramen lacerum

Figure 8 Inferior view of the cranial base. Note the fossa, foramen, meatus, groove, spine, tubercule, and process.

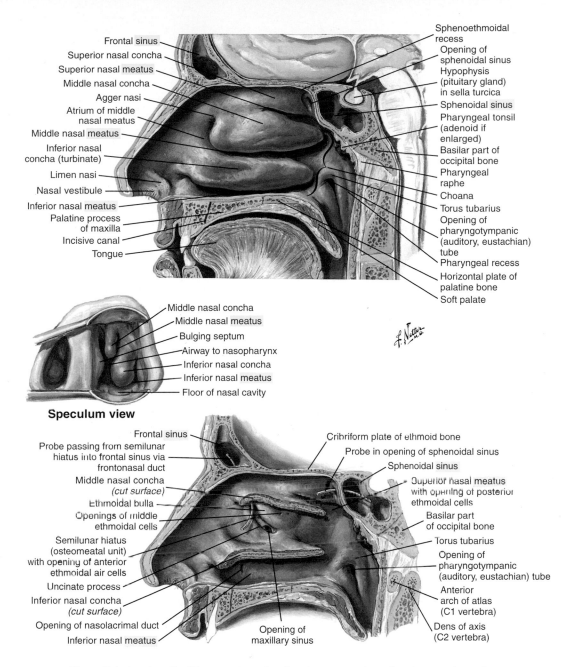

Frontal sinus
Superior nasal concha
Superior nasal meatus
Middle nasal concha
Agger nasi
Atrium of middle nasal meatus
Middle nasal meatus
Inferior nasal concha (turbinate)
Limen nasi
Nasal vestibule
Inferior nasal meatus
Palatine process of maxilla
Incisive canal
Tongue

Sphenoethmoidal recess
Opening of sphenoidal sinus
Hypophysis (pituitary gland) in sella turcica
Sphenoidal sinus
Pharyngeal tonsil (adenoid if enlarged)
Basilar part of occipital bone
Pharyngeal raphe
Choana
Torus tubarius
Opening of pharyngotympanic (auditory, eustachian) tube
Pharyngeal recess
Horizontal plate of palatine bone
Soft palate

f. Netter.

Middle nasal concha
Middle nasal meatus
Bulging septum
Airway to nasopharynx
Inferior nasal concha
Inferior nasal meatus
Floor of nasal cavity

Speculum view

Frontal sinus
Probe passing from semilunar hiatus into frontal sinus via frontonasal duct
Middle nasal concha (cut surface)
Ethmoidal bulla
Openings of middle ethmoidal cells
Semilunar hiatus (osteomeatal unit) with opening of anterior ethmoidal air cells
Uncinate process
Inferior nasal concha (cut surface)
Opening of nasolacrimal duct
Inferior nasal meatus

Cribriform plate of ethmoid bone
Probe in opening of sphenoidal sinus
Sphenoidal sinus
Superior nasal meatus with opening of posterior ethmoidal cells
Basilar part of occipital bone
Torus tubarius
Opening of pharyngotympanic (auditory, eustachian) tube
Anterior arch of atlas (C1 vertebra)
Dens of axis (C2 vertebra)

Opening of maxillary sinus

Figure 9 Lateral wall of the nasal cavity showing examples of a sinus and meatus.

Elevations

- A condyle is a rounded point of articulation (Figure 10).
- A crest is a ridge (Figure 10).
- A head is an enlargement of the extremity of a bone (Figure 10).
- A process is a prominence or extension (see Figure 8 [p. 18]).
- A protuberance is a projection beyond the surface.
- A spine is a spike-shaped projection.
- A tubercle is a small, rounded protuberance (Figure 10; see also Figure 7 [p. 17]).
- A tuberosity is a larger, rounded protuberance (Figure 10).

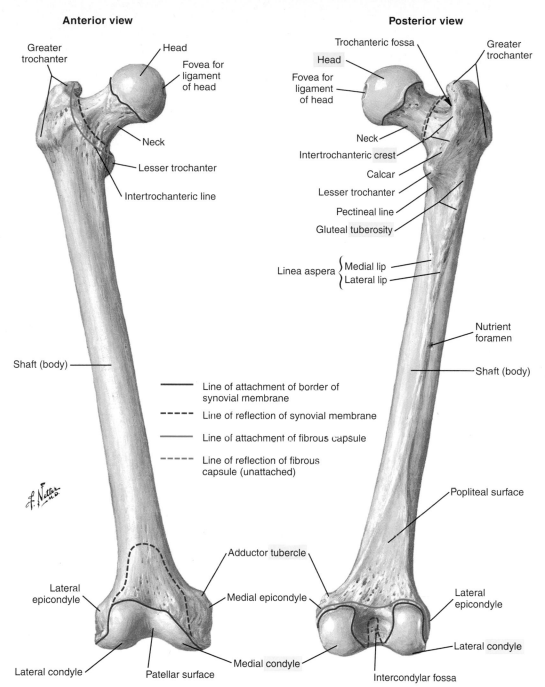

Anterior view

Greater trochanter

Head

Fovea for ligament of head

Neck

Lesser trochanter

Intertrochanteric line

Shaft (body)

—— Line of attachment of border of synovial membrane

----- Line of reflection of synovial membrane

—— Line of attachment of fibrous capsule

----- Line of reflection of fibrous capsule (unattached)

Lateral epicondyle

Adductor tubercle

Medial epicondyle

Lateral condyle

Patellar surface

Medial condyle

Posterior view

Trochanteric fossa

Greater trochanter

Head

Fovea for ligament of head

Neck

Intertrochanteric crest

Calcar

Lesser trochanter

Pectineal line

Gluteal tuberosity

Linea aspera { Medial lip
Lateral lip

Nutrient foramen

Shaft (body)

Popliteal surface

Lateral epicondyle

Lateral condyle

Intercondylar fossa

Figure 10 Anterior and posterior views of the femur. Note the condyle, crest, head, tubercle, and tuberosity.

RESPIRATORY SYSTEM

■ OVERVIEW

The respiratory system is vital for the elimination of carbon dioxide and the absorption of oxygen. Superimposed on this primary biological function is the use of the respiratory system for speech production. The respiratory system is the source of energy for vocal fold vibration and consonant production by the oral articulators. Breathing and swallowing must be well coordinated to protect the airways, and the respiratory system is also involved in airway-protective functions, such as cough.

For speech production, the pressure beneath the closed vocal folds (subglottal pressure) must be maintained within a relatively narrow range. The maintenance of a relatively constant subglottal pressure requires a complex interaction between the forces generated by the passive mechanical properties of the lungs and thorax and those generated by active muscular contraction. Even though subglottal pressure is maintained relatively constant for vocal fold vibration, it is possible to modulate this pressure up or down for changes in loudness (intensity).

Speech is produced within a relatively small range of vital capacity. During speech, inspirations usually terminate at lung volumes slightly higher than those associated with quiet breathing, and they are rapid to avoid interruptions to the flow of speech. Expirations are prolonged compared with those during quiet breathing, and because we speak during the expiratory phase, their duration, and whether they go to lung volumes below the resting expiratory level (lung volume at the end of expiration during quiet breathing), is influenced by communication demands.

Swallowing requires precise coordination with respiratory processes to ensure adequate airway protection during the passage of food and fluids, including saliva. The airways need to be protected during swallowing because the food or liquid bolus and air share a common passageway. Effective coordination helps prevent aspirations that occur when a portion of food, liquid, or saliva enters the lower respiratory tract. Airway-protective mechanisms during swallowing include vocal fold closure, anterior-superior displacement of the larynx, velopharyngeal closure, and respiratory inhibition. Swallowing typically begins in the mid to late expiratory phase of quiet breathing. This coordination is optimal for swallowing efficiency and airway protection. Cough, which is important for airway protection, involves high expiratory forces and sufficient air flow to clear the airways.

The respiratory system is the topic of Part 1, beginning with a brief overview of the skeletal support for respiration and then addressing the lungs and associated respiratory structures. Finally, respiratory muscles and their functions are reviewed.

■ SKELETAL SUPPORT FOR RESPIRATION

Skeletal support for respiration is composed of the following elements (see Figures 1.3 [p. 31] and 1.4 [p. 33]):
- Posteriorly by the vertebral column
- Anteriorly by the sternum and cartilages
- Laterally by the ribs
- Superiorly by the scapular girdle
- Inferiorly by the pelvic girdle

Vertebral Column (Figure 1.1)

The vertebral column contains 32 to 33 vertebrae that are numbered superiorly to inferiorly in 5 regions, as follows:
- 7 cervical vertebrae
- 12 thoracic vertebrae (that articulate with 12 ribs)
- 5 lumbar vertebrae
- 5 sacral vertebrae
- 3 to 4 coccygeal vertebrae

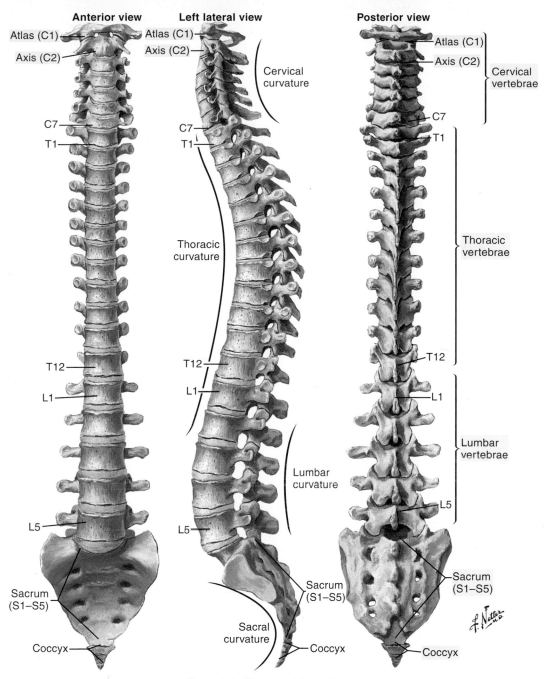

Figure 1.1. The vertebral column.

A *typical thoracic* vertebra contains the following elements (Figure 1.2):
- A vertebral body with two superior and two inferior costal facets that articulate with the head of the ribs above and below each vertebra (to *articulate* means to "come closer and form a junction").
- A vertebral foramen (canal for the spinal cord).
- Two superior and two inferior articular processes and facets where adjacent vertebrae articulate.
- Two transverse processes projecting laterally with transverse costal facets at their extremities, which articulate with the tubercle of the ribs. Transverse processes of thoracic vertebrae are points of attachment of several deep back muscles and ligaments.
- A spinous process projecting posteriorly and slightly downwards that provides a point attachment of deep and superficial muscles and ligaments of the back.

Refer to Figure 1.1 (p. 27) to see the following:
- Note the change in the form of the vertebrae. Inferior vertebrae are more massive to support more weight.
- The vertebral column contains four curves (cervical, thoracic, lumbar, and sacral). These curves give a double S shape to the vertebral column and increase its strength and flexibility to support body weight and movement.
- Two cervical vertebrae have anatomical and functional characteristics that are different from the other vertebrae. The first cervical vertebra (C1), or atlas (after Greek mythology), has no body or spinous process, supports the head, and allows for head rotation and other movements. The second cervical vertebra (C2), or axis, has an odontoid (meaning toothlike) process that serves as a pivot point for head rotation.
- The seventh cervical vertebra (C7) has a long spinous process that is often easy to locate and palpate on the skin's surface.
- Sacral vertebrae are normally fused in the adult. They reinforce and stabilize the pelvis and form the sacrum.
- Coccygeal vertebrae are also fused and form a small triangular bone, the coccyx.
- Intervertebral discs of fibrocartilage lie between adjacent vertebrae, except for between the atlas and axis and between adjacent sacral and coccygeal vertebrae (which are fused). There is a large intervertebral disc between the last lumbar (L5) and first sacral (S1) vertebrae (the lumbosacral joint) and a small, atypical disc between the last sacral (S5) and first coccygeal (Co1) vertebrae (the sacrococcygeal joint). Discs provide for movement and shock absorption.

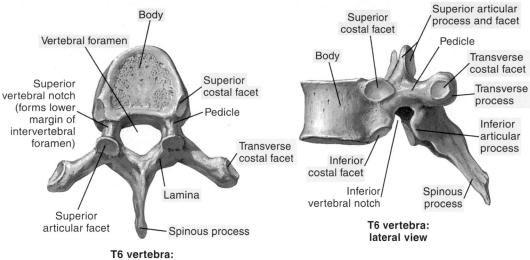

**T6 vertebra:
superior view**

**T6 vertebra:
lateral view**

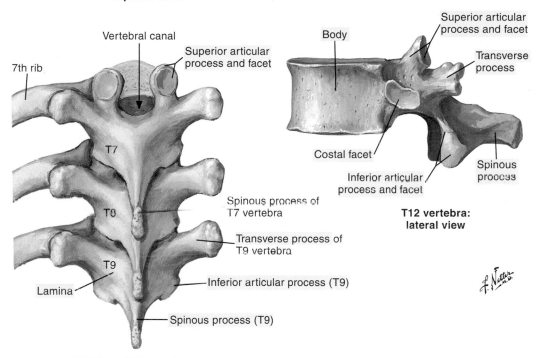

**T7, T8, and T9 vertebrae:
posterior view**

**T12 vertebra:
lateral view**

Figure 1.2. The thoracic vertebrae.

Rib Cage (Ribs, Cartilages, Sternum) (Figure 1.3)

The human body contains the following 12 pairs of ribs:

- Ribs 1 through 7 are "true" ribs (or vertebrosternal ribs) and connect directly to the sternum via costal cartilages (for mobility).
- Ribs 8, 9, and 10 are "false" ribs and connect to the sternum via a common cartilage that joins the seventh costal cartilage.
- Ribs 11 and 12 are "floating" ribs; their anterior extremity is free (not connected to the sternum).

The posterior extremity of each rib is connected to the vertebral column. The sternum is connected to the ribs and clavicles and is composed of the following three parts:

1. The manubrium
2. The body or corpus
3. The xiphoid process

The articulation of the manubrium with the corpus forms the sternal angle, or angle of Louis, and marks the approximate location of the second costal cartilages and the level of tracheal bifurcation.

Pectoral, Scapular, or Shoulder Girdle (Figure 1.3)

- The pectoral, scapular, or shoulder girdle is formed anteriorly by the clavicle (long thin bone) and posteriorly by the scapula (triangular flat bone).
- The clavicle allows for the projection of the scapula away from the thoracic cage.
- The humerus is attached to the glenoid cavity of the scapula.
- The pectoral girdle is the point of attachment for many accessory muscles of respiration such as the pectoralis major and sternocleidomastoid muscles. Fixation or stabilization of the pectoral girdle is needed for forced inspiration and expiration, as well as for heavy lifting and other strenuous activities.

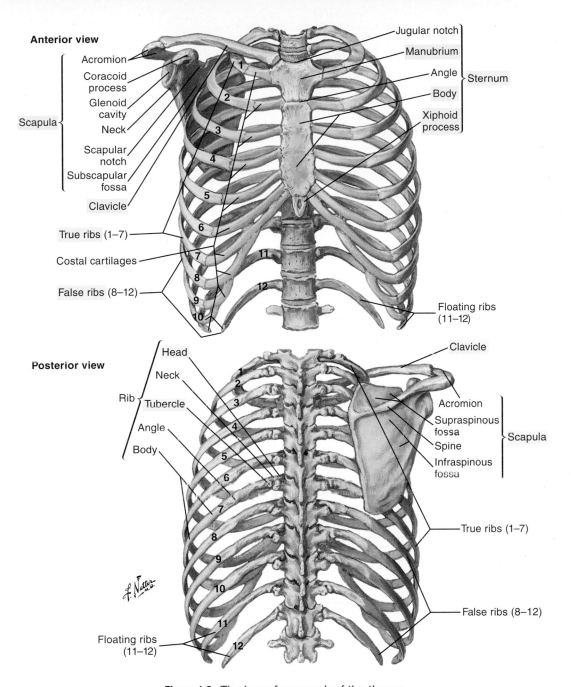

Anterior view

- Acromion
- Coracoid process
- Glenoid cavity
- Neck
- Scapular notch
- Subscapular fossa
- Clavicle
- Scapula

- Jugular notch
- Manubrium
- Angle
- Body
- Xiphoid process
- Sternum

- True ribs (1–7)
- Costal cartilages
- False ribs (8–12)
- Floating ribs (11–12)

Posterior view

- Head
- Neck
- Rib
- Tubercle
- Angle
- Body
- Floating ribs (11–12)

- Clavicle
- Acromion
- Supraspinous fossa
- Spine
- Infraspinous fossa
- Scapula
- True ribs (1–7)
- False ribs (8–12)

Figure 1.3. The bony framework of the thorax.

Pelvic Girdle or Bony Pelvis (Figure 1.4)

The pelvic girdle is formed by the following:

- A pair of symmetrical coxal, or hip, bones that are joined together anteriorly at the pubic symphysis and posteriorly by the sacrum. Each hip bone is composed of three distinct bones that fuse during development. The following individual structures retain their names despite the fact that they are fused and no suture lines may be visible:
  - Ilium
  - Ischium
  - Pubis
- The sacrum is attached to the ilium at the sacroiliac joint, an extremely strong and stable joint that supports the weight of the upper body.
- The coccyx is the final segment of the vertebral column and is often referred to as the "tailbone."

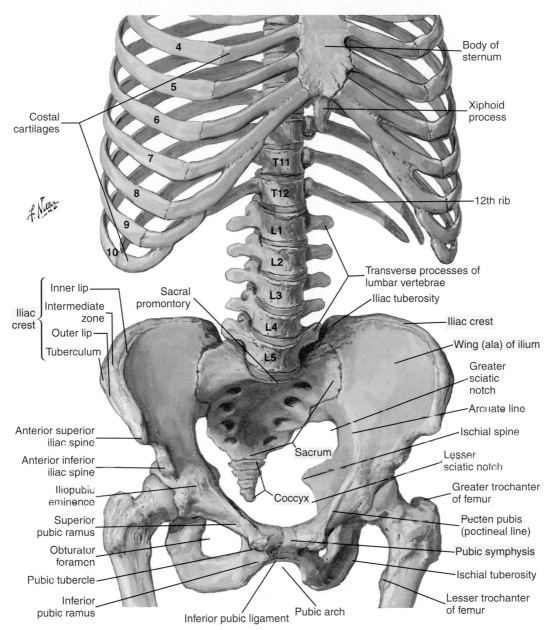

Figure 1.4. The bony framework of the abdomen.

■ RESPIRATORY TRACT

Air circulates in the following respiratory areas:
- Nasal cavity
- Oral cavity
- Pharynx
- Larynx
- Trachea
- Bronchi
- Lungs

Nasal Cavity (Figure 1.5)

The nasal cavity is the first segment of the upper respiratory tract and participates in olfaction (see Part 3: Oropharyngeal-Articulatory System, pp. 107–171).

Oral Cavity

The oral cavity is delimited anteriorly and laterally by the teeth, posteriorly by the palatoglossal arch (anterior faucial pillar), superiorly by the hard palate and soft palate, and inferiorly by the tongue. It is located posteriorly and medially to the oral vestibule (the space between the lips or the cheeks and the gums and teeth), and anteriorly to the pharynx (see Part 3: Oropharyngeal-Articulatory System, pp. 107–171).

Pharynx (Figure 1.6 [p. 36])

The pharynx is a vertically oriented, muscular passageway that provides communication between the buccal/oral cavity and the esophagus and between the nasal cavity and the larynx (see Part 3: Oropharyngeal-Articulatory System, pp. 107–171).

The pharynx is composed of the following:
- Nasopharynx (portion located behind the nasal cavity)
- Oropharynx (portion located behind the oral cavity)
- Laryngopharynx or hypopharynx (portion located behind the larynx)

Larynx (Figure 1.7 [p. 37])

The larynx is located directly above the trachea and in front of the pharynx. The principal biological function of the larynx is to protect the lower respiratory tract (see Part 2: Laryngeal-Phonatory System, pp. 77–106).

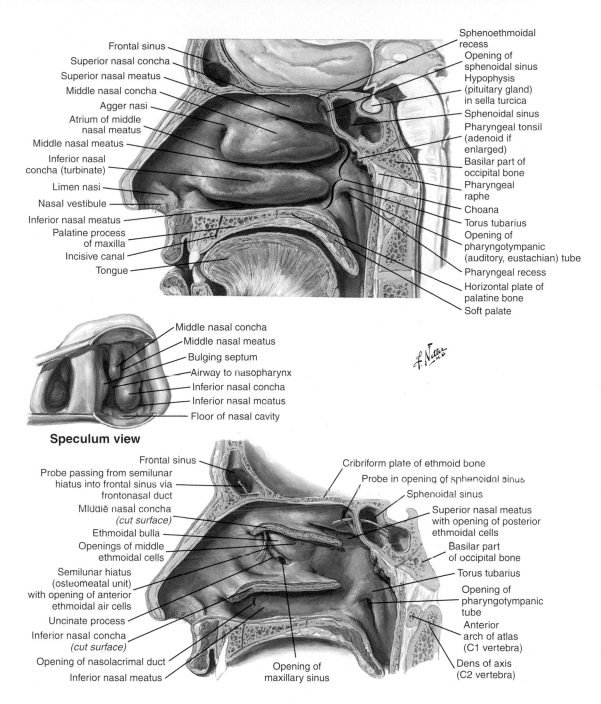

Frontal sinus
Superior nasal concha
Superior nasal meatus
Middle nasal concha
Agger nasi
Atrium of middle nasal meatus
Middle nasal meatus
Inferior nasal concha (turbinate)
Limen nasi
Nasal vestibule
Inferior nasal meatus
Palatine process of maxilla
Incisive canal
Tongue

Sphenoethmoidal recess
Opening of sphenoidal sinus
Hypophysis (pituitary gland) in sella turcica
Sphenoidal sinus
Pharyngeal tonsil (adenoid if enlarged)
Basilar part of occipital bone
Pharyngeal raphe
Choana
Torus tubarius
Opening of pharyngotympanic (auditory, eustachian) tube
Pharyngeal recess
Horizontal plate of palatine bone
Soft palate

Middle nasal concha
Middle nasal meatus
Bulging septum
Airway to nasopharynx
Inferior nasal concha
Inferior nasal meatus
Floor of nasal cavity

Speculum view

Frontal sinus
Probe passing from semilunar hiatus into frontal sinus via frontonasal duct
Middle nasal concha (cut surface)
Ethmoidal bulla
Openings of middle ethmoidal cells
Semilunar hiatus (osteomeatal unit) with opening of anterior ethmoidal air cells
Uncinate process
Inferior nasal concha (cut surface)
Opening of nasolacrimal duct
Inferior nasal meatus

Cribriform plate of ethmoid bone
Probe in opening of sphenoidal sinus
Sphenoidal sinus
Superior nasal meatus with opening of posterior ethmoidal cells
Basilar part of occipital bone
Torus tubarius
Opening of pharyngotympanic tube
Anterior arch of atlas (C1 vertebra)
Dens of axis (C2 vertebra)

Opening of maxillary sinus

Figure 1.5. The lateral wall of the nasal cavity.

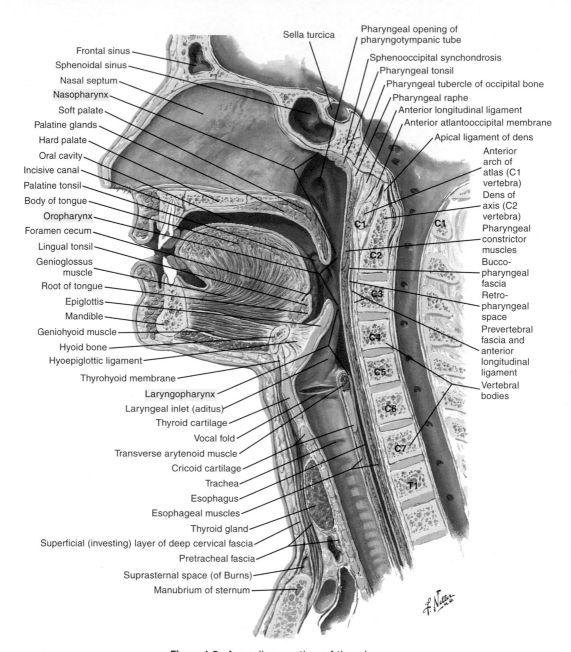

Figure 1.6. A median section of the pharynx.

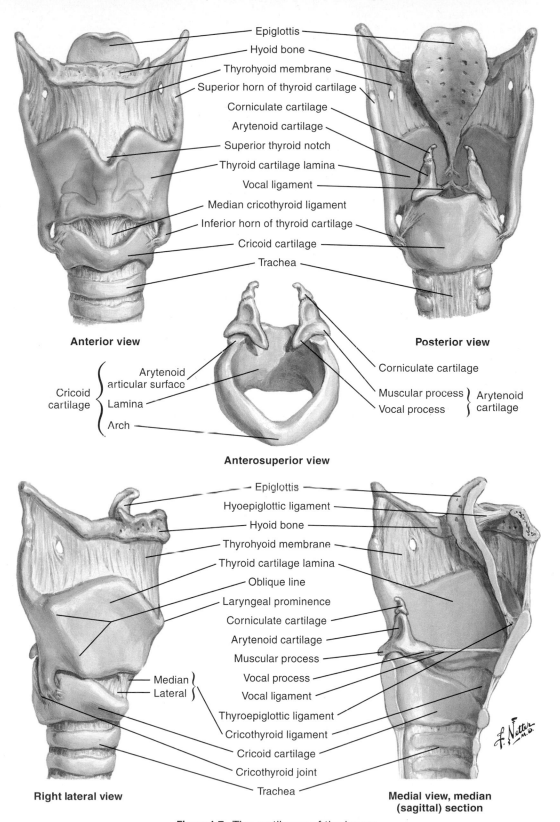

Figure 1.7. The cartilages of the larynx.

Trachea (Figure 1.8)

The trachea extends from the larynx to the bronchi. It contains 16 to 20 incomplete cartilaginous, horseshoe-shaped rings connected by ligaments. The rings are deficient posteriorly to accommodate the attachment to the esophagus. The trachea has two portions: (1) cervical and (2) thoracic.

Bronchi (Figures 1.8 and 1.9 [p. 40])

The trachea divides, or bifurcates, at the level of the sternal angle (T4 to T5) to form the main, or primary, bronchi (right and left), as follows:

- The main bronchi divide into lobar or secondary bronchi, one for each lung lobe: three for the right lung (superior, middle, and inferior) and two for the left lung (superior and inferior).
- The lobar bronchi further divide to form segmental or tertiary bronchi (third-order bronchi), each supplying a specific bronchopulmonary segment: 10 for the right and 8 to 10 for the left (depending on whether certain bronchopulmonary segments share the same segmental bronchus).
- The segmental bronchi continue to divide many times (20 to 25 generations) to eventually become terminal bronchioles ("little tubes") with diameters of less than 0.5 mm. The terminal bronchioles are the end of the conducting respiratory passageways.

The respiratory portion of the pathway in which gas exchange occurs begins with the respiratory bronchioles, then the alveolar ducts, the alveolar sacs, and the alveoli, in which the main part of pulmonary gas exchange occurs (Figure 1.10 [p. 41]).

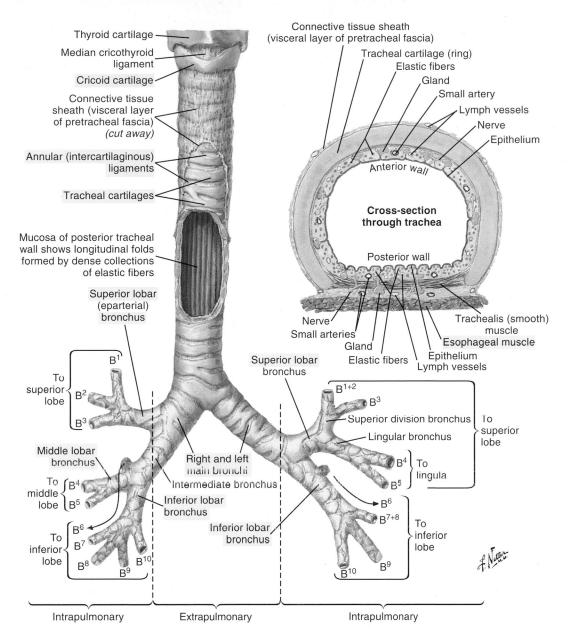

Figure 1.8. The trachea and major bronchi.

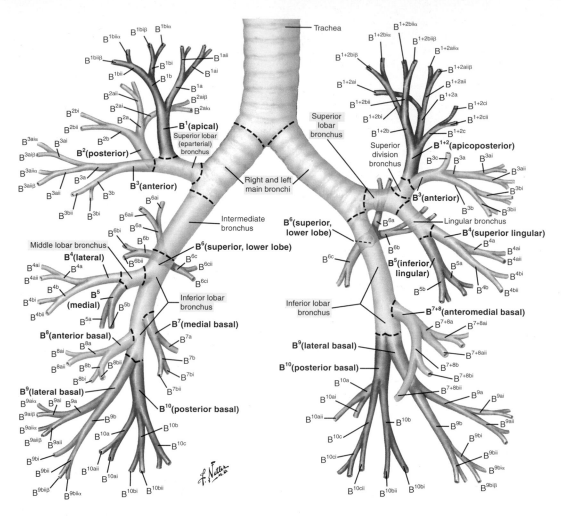

Nomenclature in common usage for bronchopulmonary segments is that of Jackson and Huber, and segmental bronchi are named accordingly. Ikeda proposed nomenclature (as demonstrated here) for bronchial subdivisions as far as 6th generation. For simplification on this illustration, only some bronchial subdivisions are labeled as far as 5th or 6th generation. Segmental bronchi (B) are numbered from 1 to 10 in each lung, corresponding to pulmonary segments. In left lung, B[1] and B[2] are combined,

as are B[7] and B[8]. Subsegmental, or 4th order, bronchi are indicated by addition of lower-case letters a, b, or c when an additional branch is present. Fifth order bronchi are designated by Roman numerals i (anterior) or ii (posterior) and 6th order bronchi by Greek letters α or β. Several texts use alternate numbers (as proposed by Boyden) for segmental bronchi.

Variations of standard bronchial pattern shown here are common, especially in peripheral airways.

Figure 1.9. The nomenclature of the bronchi.

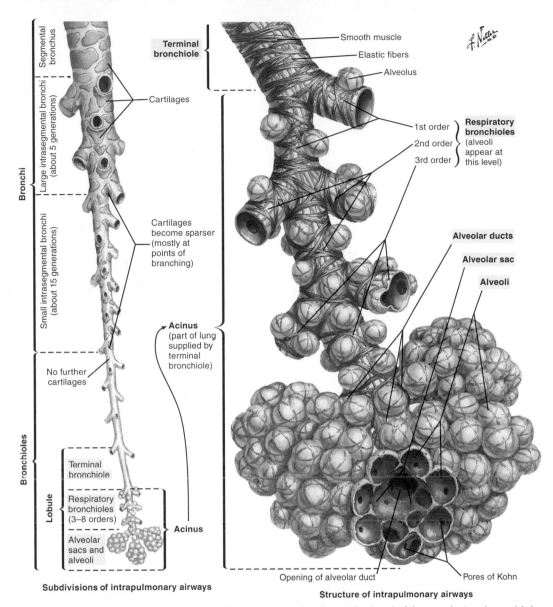

Terminal bronchiole

Cartilages

Cartilages become sparser (mostly at points of branching)

Acinus (part of lung supplied by terminal bronchiole)

No further cartilages

Segmental bronchus

Large intrasegmental bronchi (about 5 generations)

Small intrasegmental bronchi (about 15 generations)

Bronchi

Bronchioles

Lobule

Terminal bronchiole

Respiratory bronchioles (3–8 orders)

Alveolar sacs and alveoli

Acinus

Subdivisions of intrapulmonary airways

Smooth muscle

Elastic fibers

Alveolus

1st order

2nd order

3rd order

Respiratory bronchioles (alveoli appear at this level)

Alveolar ducts

Alveolar sac

Alveoli

Opening of alveolar duct

Pores of Kohn

Structure of intrapulmonary airways

Figure 1.10. The intrapulmonary airways. Gas exchange begins at the level of the respiratory bronchioles.

Lungs (Figure 1.11)

The trunk, or torso, contains the thorax (or thoracic cavity) and the abdomen, which are divided by the diaphragm. The lungs are located in the thorax. They are two masses of non-muscular tissue that occupy a major portion of the thoracic cavity. Between the right and left lungs is a space called the *mediastinum* that contains the heart and other anatomical structures (Figure 1.12 [p. 44]).

The lungs are spongy, porous, and highly elastic. Because they are elastic, they seek to return to their relaxed or resting position when stretched or compressed.

Although similar in appearance and function, the following differences in the shape of the two lungs are a result of the presence of adjacent organs (Figure 1.13 [p. 45]):

- The right lung is larger and broader than the left but shorter because of the presence of the liver and the elevation of the diaphragm on the right side. The overall capacity and weight of the right lung are greater than those of the left.
- The left lung is smaller and narrower than the right lung, with a distinct cardiac notch to accommodate the pericardium (membrane covering the heart and great blood vessels).
- The right lung is divided into three lobes by the horizontal (minor) and oblique (major) fissures.
- The left lung is divided into two lobes by an oblique fissure (major fissure).
- Each lung is anatomically divided into functional segments called *bronchopulmonary segments* (10 for the right and 8 to 10 for the left).
- The superior aspect of each lung is called the *apex,* and the inferior aspect is called the *base.*
- Each lung has an inferior concave diaphragmatic surface, an external convex costal surface, and an internal concave surface that is caused by the presence of the mediastinum.
- The lung apex can exceed the limits of the thorax and protrude above the level of the middle third of the clavicle by several centimeters.

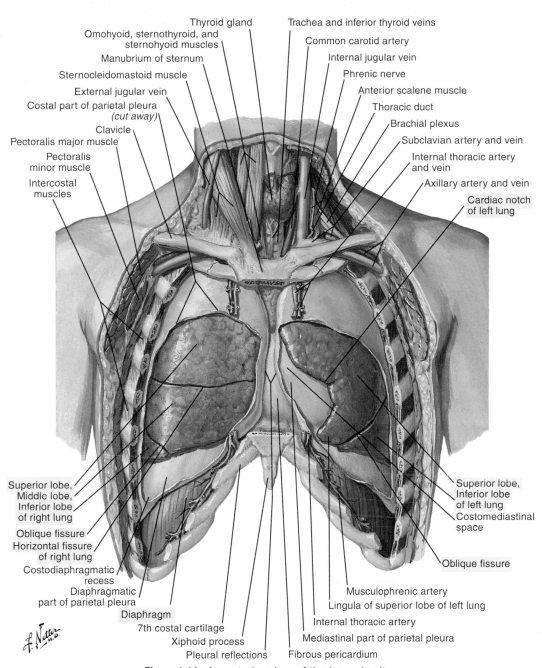

Thyroid gland
Omohyoid, sternothyroid, and sternohyoid muscles
Manubrium of sternum
Sternocleidomastoid muscle
External jugular vein
Costal part of parietal pleura *(cut away)*
Clavicle
Pectoralis major muscle
Pectoralis minor muscle
Intercostal muscles

Trachea and inferior thyroid veins
Common carotid artery
Internal jugular vein
Phrenic nerve
Anterior scalene muscle
Thoracic duct
Brachial plexus
Subclavian artery and vein
Internal thoracic artery and vein
Axillary artery and vein
Cardiac notch of left lung

Superior lobe,
Middle lobe,
Inferior lobe
of right lung
Oblique fissure
Horizontal fissure of right lung
Costodiaphragmatic recess
Diaphragmatic part of parietal pleura
Diaphragm
7th costal cartilage
Xiphoid process
Pleural reflections

Superior lobe,
Inferior lobe
of left lung
Costomediastinal space
Oblique fissure

Musculophrenic artery
Lingula of superior lobe of left lung
Internal thoracic artery
Mediastinal part of parietal pleura
Fibrous pericardium

Figure 1.11. An anterior view of the lungs in situ.

Phrenic Nerve

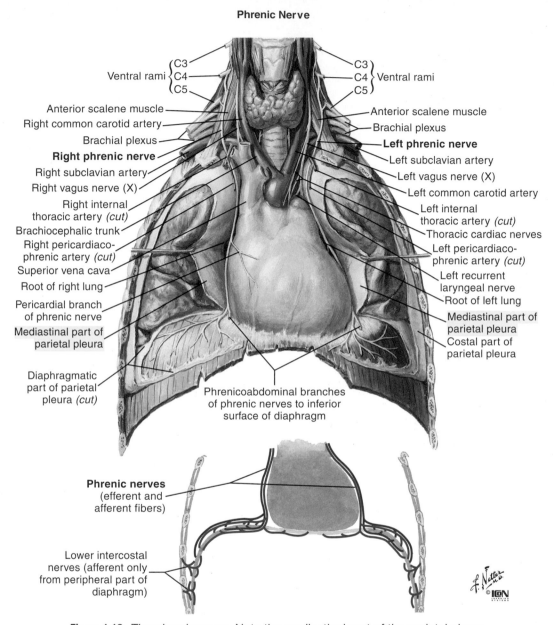

C3
Ventral rami { C4
C5

C3
C4 } Ventral rami
C5

Anterior scalene muscle
Right common carotid artery
Brachial plexus
Right phrenic nerve
Right subclavian artery
Right vagus nerve (X)
Right internal thoracic artery *(cut)*
Brachiocephalic trunk
Right pericardiaco-phrenic artery *(cut)*
Superior vena cava
Root of right lung
Pericardial branch of phrenic nerve
Mediastinal part of parietal pleura
Diaphragmatic part of parietal pleura *(cut)*

Anterior scalene muscle
Brachial plexus
Left phrenic nerve
Left subclavian artery
Left vagus nerve (X)
Left common carotid artery
Left internal thoracic artery *(cut)*
Thoracic cardiac nerves
Left pericardiaco-phrenic artery *(cut)*
Left recurrent laryngeal nerve
Root of left lung
Mediastinal part of parietal pleura
Costal part of parietal pleura

Phrenicoabdominal branches of phrenic nerves to inferior surface of diaphragm

Phrenic nerves (efferent and afferent fibers)

Lower intercostal nerves (afferent only from peripheral part of diaphragm)

Figure 1.12. The phrenic nerve. Note the mediastinal part of the parietal pleura.

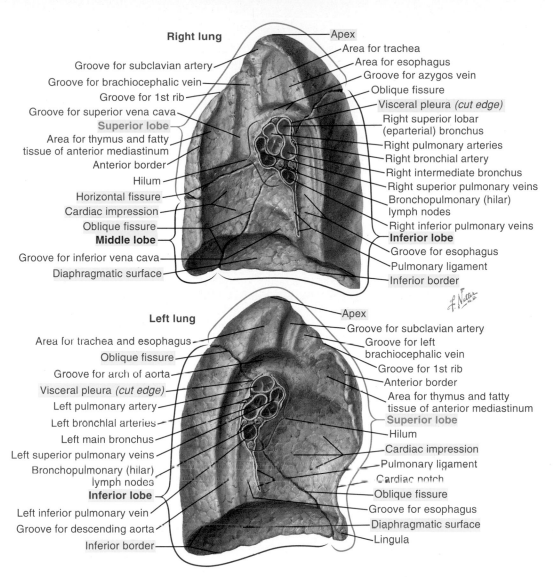

Right lung

Groove for subclavian artery
Groove for brachiocephalic vein
Groove for 1st rib
Groove for superior vena cava
Superior lobe
Area for thymus and fatty tissue of anterior mediastinum
Anterior border
Hilum
Horizontal fissure
Cardiac impression
Oblique fissure
Middle lobe
Groove for inferior vena cava
Diaphragmatic surface

Apex
Area for trachea
Area for esophagus
Groove for azygos vein
Oblique fissure
Visceral pleura (cut edge)
Right superior lobar (eparterial) bronchus
Right pulmonary arteries
Right bronchial artery
Right intermediate bronchus
Right superior pulmonary veins
Bronchopulmonary (hilar) lymph nodes
Right inferior pulmonary veins
Inferior lobe
Groove for esophagus
Pulmonary ligament
Inferior border

Left lung

Area for trachea and esophagus
Oblique fissure
Groove for arch of aorta
Visceral pleura (cut edge)
Left pulmonary artery
Left bronchial arteries
Left main bronchus
Left superior pulmonary veins
Bronchopulmonary (hilar) lymph nodes
Inferior lobe
Left inferior pulmonary vein
Groove for descending aorta
Inferior border

Apex
Groove for subclavian artery
Groove for left brachiocephalic vein
Groove for 1st rib
Anterior border
Area for thymus and fatty tissue of anterior mediastinum
Superior lobe
Hilum
Cardiac impression
Pulmonary ligament
Cardiac notch
Oblique fissure
Groove for esophagus
Diaphragmatic surface
Lingula

Figure 1.13. Medial views of the right and left lungs.

Pleura (Figure 1.14)

The pleurae are intrathoracic serous membranes that envelop and protect the lungs:
- The parietal pleurae line the inner surface of the thoracic cavity.
- The visceral pleurae cover each lung independently (see Figure 1.13 [p. 45]).

Parietal and visceral pleurae are attached (linked) through a very thin, fluid-filled space called the pleural space. Fluid in the space allows for friction-free movement between the two membranes and creates surface tension and negative pressure that link the two pleurae. Respiratory muscles act to change the dimensions of the thoracic cavity, and because of pleural linkage, the volume of the lungs. This is important because the lungs are not muscular, and the only way to change their volume is by activating respiratory muscles. The lungs and thorax form a unit, the lungs-thorax unit. It is an elastic system whose point of equilibrium is at resting expiratory level (REL). If the lungs-thorax unit is moved away from its resting, equilibrium state at REL (by the action of inspiratory or expiratory muscles), recoil forces are generated. To illustrate these forces, imagine stretching an elastic band between your two fingers and "feeling" the tension acting to return the elastic to its starting (unstretched) position. Or imagine compressing a sponge in your hands and "feeling" a force working to return the sponge to its uncompressed state. These forces generate what we call *relaxation pressures,* which are important components for quiet breathing and for speech.

Selected Pulmonary Disorders Affecting Lung Function

- **Pleurisy** is an inflammation of the pleura caused by an undersecretion or oversecretion of fluid in the pleural space. Respiration may be very painful.
- **Pneumothorax** is the presence of air in the pleural space (the result of trauma such as a penetrating chest wound or disease). This condition may interrupt pleural linkage and cause a collapse of one or both of the lungs, depending on whether the pneumothorax is unilateral or bilateral.
- **Pneumonia** is an infection of the lungs resulting from many possible causes, including the presence of bacteria, viruses, and fungi. Pneumonia may be the result of disordered swallowing and the aspiration (breathing in) of food and liquids. This is referred to as *aspiration pneumonia.*

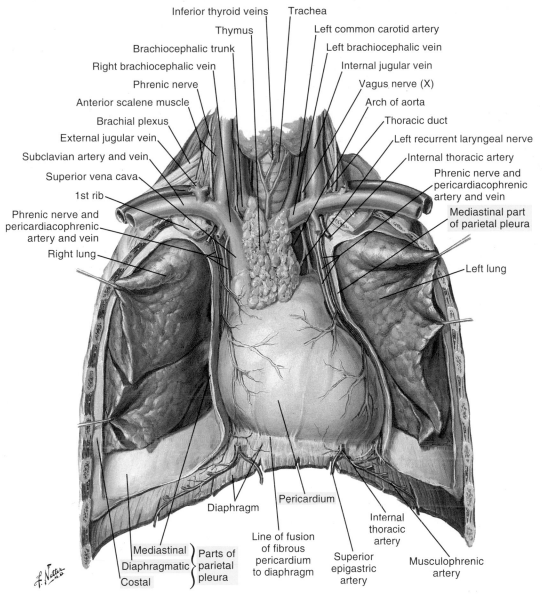

Inferior thyroid veins
Thymus
Brachiocephalic trunk
Right brachiocephalic vein
Phrenic nerve
Anterior scalene muscle
Brachial plexus
External jugular vein
Subclavian artery and vein
Superior vena cava
1st rib
Phrenic nerve and pericardiacophrenic artery and vein
Right lung

Trachea
Left common carotid artery
Left brachiocephalic vein
Internal jugular vein
Vagus nerve (X)
Arch of aorta
Thoracic duct
Left recurrent laryngeal nerve
Internal thoracic artery
Phrenic nerve and pericardiacophrenic artery and vein
Mediastinal part of parietal pleura
Left lung

Diaphragm
Pericardium

Mediastinal
Diaphragmatic } Parts of parietal pleura
Costal

Line of fusion of fibrous pericardium to diaphragm
Superior epigastric artery
Internal thoracic artery
Musculophrenic artery

Figure 1.14. The heart in situ. Note the parts of the parietal pleura.

■ RESPIRATORY MUSCLES

A very large number of muscles are potentially involved in respiration. Our focus here is on the principal muscles of respiration, which are classified as either inspiratory or expiratory (see the tables on pp. 67, 68, and 70). This historical classification is based on the isolated action of each muscle. Inspiratory muscles are those muscles whose mechanical advantage or action is to increase lung volume, and expiratory muscles are those whose mechanical advantage or action is to decrease lung volume. However, it is important to note that inspiratory muscles are not solely active during inspiration and expiratory muscles are not solely active during expiration. For example, during the expiratory phase of quiet breathing, the activation of the diaphragm (a major muscle of inspiration) gradually decreases to slow recoil forces (explained earlier) of the lungs-thorax unit, acting to bring it back to its equilibrium point at REL. This allows the expiratory phase to be prolonged to ensure optimal gas exchange.

Therefore the muscles grouped in the category "inspiratory muscles" are those whose isolated action is to increase lung volume, and "expiratory muscles" are those whose isolated action is to decrease lung volume.

Principal Muscles of Inspiration

The function of the principal muscles of inspiration is to increase pulmonary volume.

Diaphragm (Figures 1.15 [p. 51], 1.16 [p. 52], and 1.17 [p. 53])

The diaphragm is an unpaired muscle. It is a thin, dome-shaped muscle with a strong central tendon (aponeurosis) and separates the thorax from the abdomen. The right part of the dome is slightly higher than the left one because of the presence of the liver. Several important structures pass through the diaphragm, including the esophagus, aorta, and major veins through the following:

- Aortic hiatus. The aorta passes behind the medial arcuate ligament and through an osseoaponeurotic opening, and thus technically does not pierce the diaphragm. This ensures that muscular contractions of the diaphragm do not affect blood flow.
- Esophageal hiatus.
- Vena cava foramen (caval opening).

The three main groups of muscle fibers, named according to their principal points of origin, are as follows:

1. The **costal part** originates from the inferior and inner surfaces of the costal cartilages and adjacent portions of the last six ribs and courses directly upward to insert into the central tendon. Costal diaphragm muscle fibers are directly apposed to the inner surface of the rib cage for approximately 6 to 9 cm through the "zone of apposition."
2. The **sternal part** originates from the inner inferior surface of the xiphoid process of the sternum and courses upward to insert into the central tendon.
3. The **lumbar** (vertebral) **part** originates from the upper lumbar vertebrae through two groups of fibers called *crura* and from the medial and lateral arcuate ligaments. Fibers course upward to insert into the central tendon.

The orientation of the fibers of the diaphragm can be visualized by imagining the fibers forming the inner walls of a bowl.

Isolated diaphragm contraction—for example, during quiet breathing—shortens its muscle fibers and pulls down on the central tendon, which increases the vertical dimensions of the lungs-thorax unit. Because of the apposition of its costal fibers on the inner inferior surface of the rib cage, the lowering of the diaphragm that meets the resistance of the abdominal contents lifts the ribs and rotates them outward, which increases the anterolateral dimensions of the rib cage. Lung volume increases, thus creating negative (inspiratory) alveolar (lung) pressure. The contraction of the diaphragm compresses the viscera and increases abdominal pressure.

When the diaphragm relaxes, it returns to its resting form, thus decreasing the vertical dimensions of the lungs-thorax unit. The ribs also rotate downward and inward, decreasing circumferential dimensions.

During quiet breathing, the diaphragm moves about 1.5 cm, while a forced inspiration (maximum inspiration) causes a displacement up to 10 cm.

By the pleural linkage between the lungs and the diaphragm, diaphragm contraction exerts a downward pull on the trachea and larynx. This traction is counterbalanced by the action of the suprahyoid muscles (see Part 2: Laryngeal-Phonatory System, p. 100) in order to stabilize the position of the larynx during quiet breathing.

The diaphragm is innervated by the phrenic nerve, which arises from cervical spinal nerves C3 to C5.

A primary function of the intercostal (internal and external) muscles is to stiffen the rib intercostal spaces and thus the chest wall. This function prevents chest wall collapse (being "sucked" in or out) when, for example during inspiration, diaphragmatic contraction generates negative intrathoracic pressures.

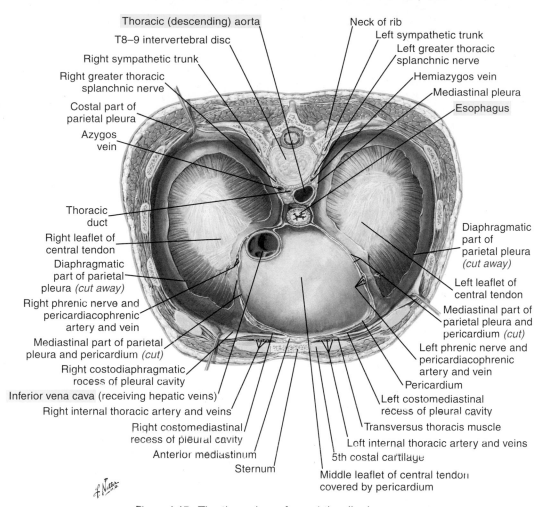

Thoracic (descending) aorta

T8–9 intervertebral disc

Right sympathetic trunk

Right greater thoracic
splanchnic nerve

Costal part of
parietal pleura

Azygos
vein

Thoracic
duct

Right leaflet of
central tendon

Diaphragmatic
part of parietal
pleura (cut away)

Right phrenic nerve and
pericardiacophrenic
artery and vein

Mediastinal part of parietal
pleura and pericardium (cut)

Right costodiaphragmatic
recess of pleural cavity

Inferior vena cava (receiving hepatic veins)

Right internal thoracic artery and veins

Right costomediastinal
recess of pleural cavity

Anterior mediastinum

Sternum

Neck of rib

Left sympathetic trunk

Left greater thoracic
splanchnic nerve

Hemiazygos vein

Mediastinal pleura

Esophagus

Diaphragmatic
part of
parietal pleura
(cut away)

Left leaflet of
central tendon

Mediastinal part of
parietal pleura and
pericardium (cut)

Left phrenic nerve and
pericardiacophrenic
artery and vein

Pericardium

Left costomediastinal
recess of pleural cavity

Transversus thoracis muscle

Left internal thoracic artery and veins

5th costal cartilage

Middle leaflet of central tendon
covered by pericardium

Figure 1.15. The thoracic surface of the diaphragm.

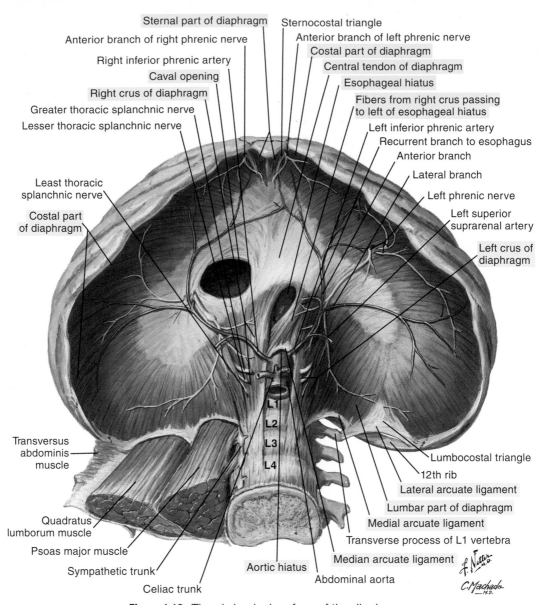

Figure 1.16. The abdominal surface of the diaphragm.

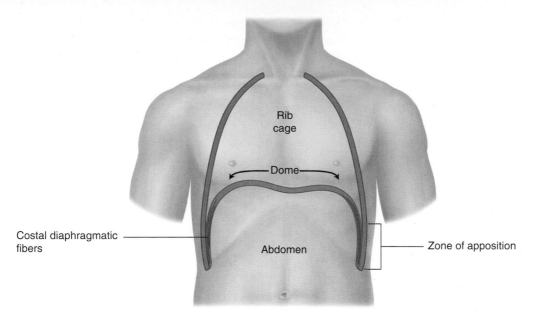

Figure 1.17. Schematic representation of the rib cage and diaphragm. Note the zone of apposition of the diaphragm. (Source: © Éléonore Lamoglia.)

External Intercostal Muscles *(Figures 1.18, 1.19 [p. 56], and 1.20 [p. 57])*

Fibers extend from the tubercles of the ribs to the junctions of the costal cartilages and the bony ribs (the costochondral junctions). From there, they are replaced by external intercostal membranes. A posterior view of the external intercostals reveals that the muscle fibers are oriented inferiorly and laterally (see Figure 1.18). Anteriorly, the muscle fibers are oriented inferiorly and medially (see Figure 1.19 [p. 56]).

There appears to be some regional distribution of the respiratory function of the external and internal intercostals (see next section). The muscle fibers located in more rostral interspaces are inspiratory, and the muscle fibers located in ventral caudal interspaces are expiratory. Inspiratory action raises the rib below; expiratory action lowers the rib above.

The external intercostal muscles are innervated by the intercostal nerves (anterior ramifications of spinal nerves T1 to T11).

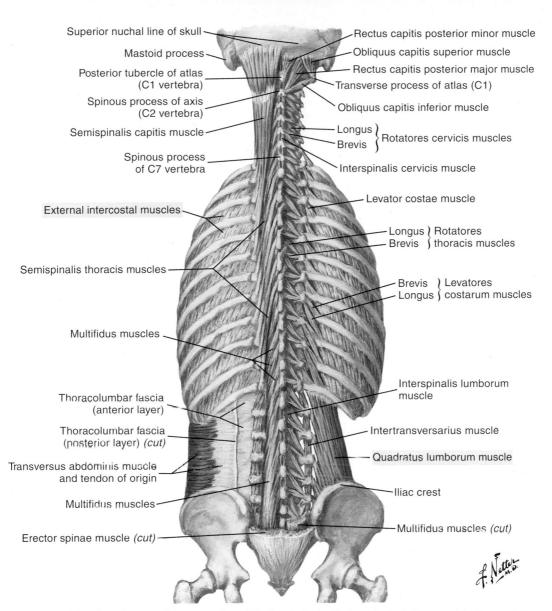

Superior nuchal line of skull

Mastoid process

Posterior tubercle of atlas
(C1 vertebra)

Spinous process of axis
(C2 vertebra)

Semispinalis capitis muscle

Spinous process
of C7 vertebra

External intercostal muscles

Semispinalis thoracis muscles

Multifidus muscles

Thoracolumbar fascia
(anterior layer)

Thoracolumbar fascia
(posterior layer) (cut)

Transversus abdominis muscle
and tendon of origin

Multifidus muscles

Erector spinae muscle (cut)

Rectus capitis posterior minor muscle

Obliquus capitis superior muscle

Rectus capitis posterior major muscle

Transverse process of atlas (C1)

Obliquus capitis inferior muscle

Longus   } Rotatores cervicis muscles
Brevis

Interspinalis cervicis muscle

Levator costae muscle

Longus } Rotatores
Brevis } thoracis muscles

Brevis } Levatores
Longus } costarum muscles

Interspinalis lumborum
muscle

Intertransversarius muscle

Quadratus lumborum muscle

Iliac crest

Multifidus muscles (cut)

Figure 1.18. The deep layers of the muscles of the back. Note that posteriorly the muscle fibers of the external intercostals are oriented inferiorly and laterally.

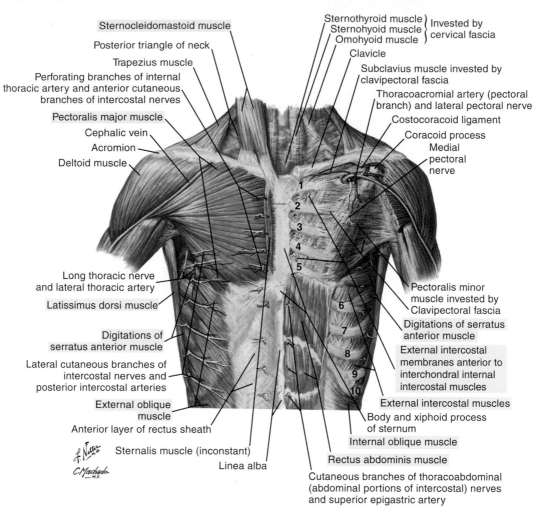

Figure 1.19. The anterior thoracic wall. Note that anteriorly the muscle fibers of the external intercostals are oriented inferiorly and medially.

Posterior and Lateral Thoracic Walls

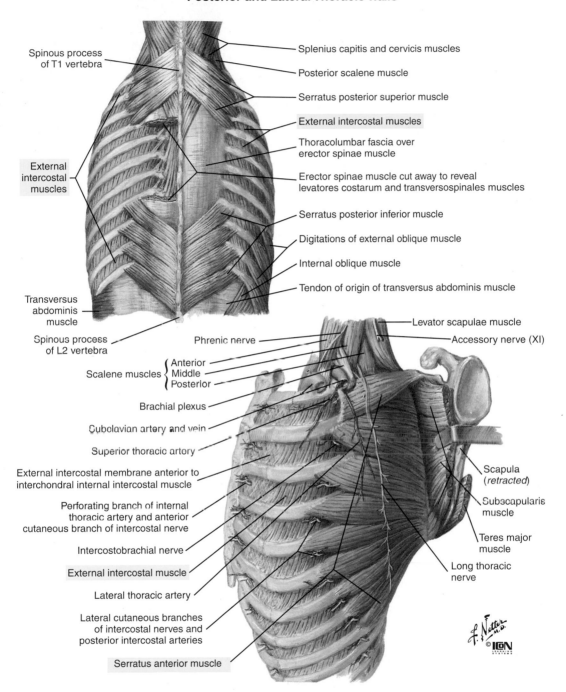

Spinous process of T1 vertebra

Splenius capitis and cervicis muscles

Posterior scalene muscle

Serratus posterior superior muscle

External intercostal muscles

Thoracolumbar fascia over erector spinae muscle

External intercostal muscles

Erector spinae muscle cut away to reveal levatores costarum and transversospinales muscles

Serratus posterior inferior muscle

Digitations of external oblique muscle

Internal oblique muscle

Tendon of origin of transversus abdominis muscle

Transversus abdominis muscle

Spinous process of L2 vertebra

Phrenic nerve

Levator scapulae muscle

Accessory nerve (XI)

Scalene muscles { Anterior / Middle / Posterior }

Brachial plexus

Subclavian artery and vein

Superior thoracic artery

Scapula (retracted)

Subscapularis muscle

External intercostal membrane anterior to interchondral internal intercostal muscle

Perforating branch of internal thoracic artery and anterior cutaneous branch of intercostal nerve

Teres major muscle

Intercostobrachial nerve

Long thoracic nerve

External intercostal muscle

Lateral thoracic artery

Lateral cutaneous branches of intercostal nerves and posterior intercostal arteries

Serratus anterior muscle

Figure 1.20. The posterior and lateral thoracic walls. Note the external intercostal muscles.

Interchondral (Parasternal) Portion of Internal Intercostal Muscles (Figures 1.21 and 1.22 [p. 61])

Fibers extend from the costochondral junction and at approximately right angles to the fibers of the external intercostals (which are absent here) to the sternum; their action is to raise the rib below.

The interchondral internal intercostals are innervated by the intercostal nerves (anterior ramifications of spinal nerves T1 to T11).

Accessory Muscles of Inspiration (Figures 1.21 and 1.22 [p. 61]; see also Figures 1.18 [p. 55], 1.19 [p. 56], and 1.20 [p. 57])

Accessory muscles of inspiration include a potentially large number of muscles that could have an inspiratory effect on the thorax and lungs. The exact respiratory function, however, of these muscles is not completely understood. For example, serratus posterior superior and levatores costarum could, via their mechanical advantage, act to elevate the ribs, but conclusive evidence of their activity during respiratory efforts is lacking.

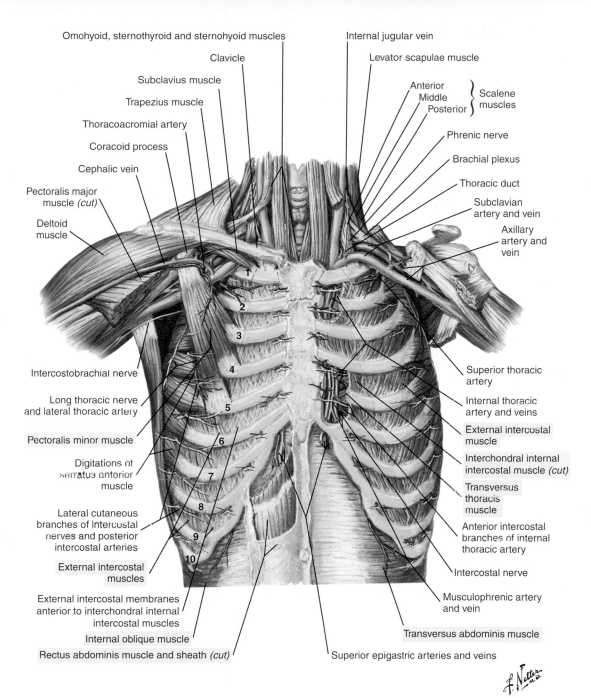

Omohyoid, sternothyroid and sternohyoid muscles

Clavicle

Subclavius muscle

Trapezius muscle

Thoracoacromial artery

Coracoid process

Cephalic vein

Pectoralis major
muscle *(cut)*

Deltoid
muscle

Intercostobrachial nerve

Long thoracic nerve
and lateral thoracic artery

Pectoralis minor muscle

Digitations of
serratus anterior
muscle

Lateral cutaneous
branches of intercostal
nerves and posterior
intercostal arteries

External intercostal
muscles

External intercostal membranes
anterior to interchondral internal
intercostal muscles

Internal oblique muscle

Rectus abdominis muscle and sheath *(cut)*

Internal jugular vein

Levator scapulae muscle

Anterior
Middle   } Scalene
Posterior   } muscles

Phrenic nerve

Brachial plexus

Thoracic duct

Subclavian
artery and vein

Axillary
artery and
vein

Superior thoracic
artery

Internal thoracic
artery and veins

External intercostal
muscle

Interchondral internal
intercostal muscle *(cut)*

Transversus
thoracis
muscle

Anterior intercostal
branches of internal
thoracic artery

Intercostal nerve

Musculophrenic artery
and vein

Transversus abdominis muscle

Superior epigastric arteries and veins

Figure 1.21. The anterior thoracic wall. Note the interchondral portion of the internal intercostal muscles.

Principal Muscles of Expiration

The function of the muscles of expiration is to decrease lung volume.

Interosseous Portion of Internal Intercostal Muscles (Figures 1.22 and 1.24 [p. 63])

Fibers extend anteriorly from the costochondral junction to near the angle of the ribs posteriorly. From there, they are replaced by the internal intercostal membrane. Located deep to the external intercostals on the inner surface of the ribs, they travel obliquely and form approximately a right angle with the external intercostals. Their action is to lower the rib above.

The interosseous internal intercostals are innervated by the intercostal nerves (anterior ramifications of spinal nerves T1 to T11).

Rectus Abdominis Muscle (Figures 1.22 and 1.23 [p. 62]; see also Figure 1.19 [p. 56])

The rectus abdominis muscle is formed by large vertical, paired muscles that extend from the pubis to the sternum and the costal cartilages of ribs 5 through 7. These parallel muscles are enclosed in the rectus sheath, which is a continuation of the abdominal aponeurosis of the more laterally located abdominal muscles. The linea alba ("white line") of this sheath separates the right and left muscles. Muscular contraction compresses the abdomen.

The rectus abdominis muscle is innervated by intercostal nerves T7 to T11 and the subcostal nerve of T12.

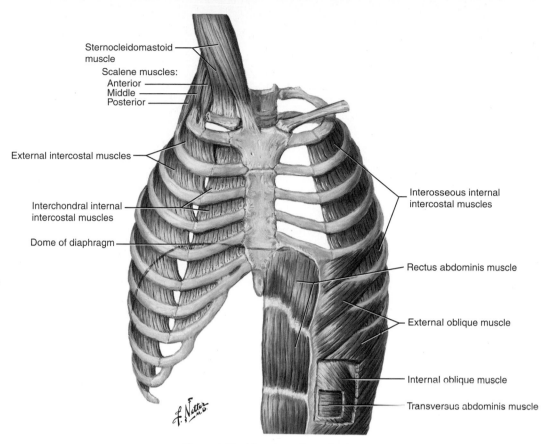

Figure 1.22. Muscles of respiration.

Sternocleidomastoid muscle

Scalene muscles:
Anterior
Middle
Posterior

External intercostal muscles

Interchondral internal intercostal muscles

Dome of diaphragm

Interosseous internal intercostal muscles

Rectus abdominis muscle

External oblique muscle

Internal oblique muscle

Transversus abdominis muscle

Lateral Views

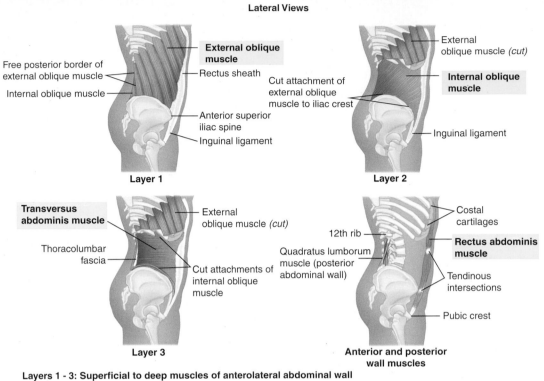

Free posterior border of external oblique muscle

Internal oblique muscle

External oblique muscle

Rectus sheath

Cut attachment of external oblique muscle to iliac crest

Anterior superior iliac spine

Inguinal ligament

Layer 1

External oblique muscle *(cut)*

Internal oblique muscle

Inguinal ligament

Layer 2

Transversus abdominis muscle

Thoracolumbar fascia

External oblique muscle *(cut)*

Cut attachments of internal oblique muscle

Layer 3

12th rib

Quadratus lumborum muscle (posterior abdominal wall)

Costal cartilages

Rectus abdominis muscle

Tendinous intersections

Pubic crest

Anterior and posterior wall muscles

Layers 1 - 3: Superficial to deep muscles of anterolateral abdominal wall

Figure 1.23. Lateral view of abdominal muscles.

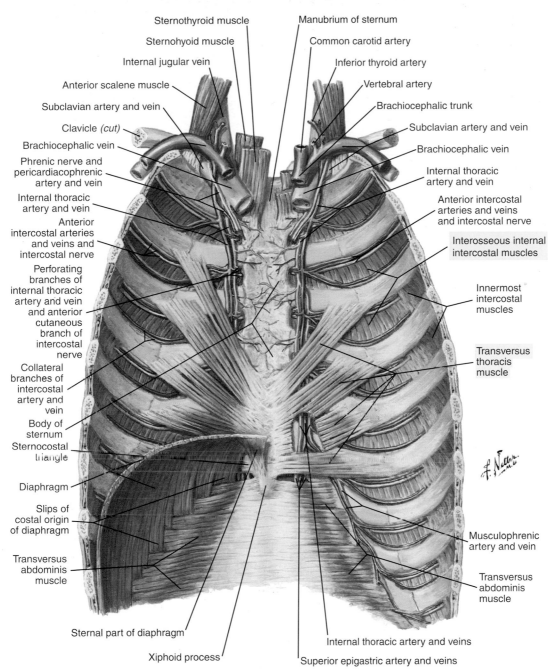

Sternothyroid muscle

Sternohyoid muscle

Internal jugular vein

Anterior scalene muscle

Subclavian artery and vein

Clavicle (cut)

Brachiocephalic vein

Phrenic nerve and pericardiacophrenic artery and vein

Internal thoracic artery and vein

Anterior intercostal arteries and veins and intercostal nerve

Perforating branches of internal thoracic artery and vein and anterior cutaneous branch of intercostal nerve

Collateral branches of intercostal artery and vein

Body of sternum

Sternocostal triangle

Diaphragm

Slips of costal origin of diaphragm

Transversus abdominis muscle

Manubrium of sternum

Common carotid artery

Inferior thyroid artery

Vertebral artery

Brachiocephalic trunk

Subclavian artery and vein

Brachiocephalic vein

Internal thoracic artery and vein

Anterior intercostal arteries and veins and intercostal nerve

Interosseous internal intercostal muscles

Innermost intercostal muscles

Transversus thoracis muscle

Musculophrenic artery and vein

Transversus abdominis muscle

Sternal part of diaphragm

Xiphoid process

Internal thoracic artery and veins

Superior epigastric artery and veins

Figure 1.24. An internal view of the anterior thoracic wall. Note the interosseous portion of the internal intercostal muscles.

External Oblique Muscle *(Figures 1.25 and 1.26 [p. 66]; see also Figures 1.19 [p. 56], 1.22 [p. 61], and 1.23 [p. 62])*

The external oblique muscle is a large sheetlike muscle that extends from the external surfaces of ribs 5 through 12. It travels obliquely medially and inferiorly to insert on the iliac crest, the inguinal ligament, and the aponeurosis of the external oblique muscle.

The external oblique muscle is innervated by intercostal nerves T7 to T11 and the subcostal nerve of T12.

Internal Oblique Muscle *(Figure 1.26 [p. 66]; see also Figures 1.19 [p. 56], 1.22 [p. 61], and 1.23 [p. 62])*

The internal oblique muscle is another sheetlike muscle that lies deep and almost perpendicular to the external oblique muscle. Fibers originate from the iliac crest, the inguinal ligament, and the thoracolumbar fascia (lumbodorsal fascia) and insert on the inferior borders of ribs 10 to 12 and the abdominal aponeurosis of the internal oblique muscle.

The internal oblique muscle is innervated by intercostal nerves T7 to T11, the subcostal nerve of T12, and the iliohypogastric and ilioinguinal branches of the first lumbar nerve.

Transversus Abdominis Muscle *(see Figures 1.21 [p. 59], 1.22 [p. 61], and 1.23 [p. 62])*

The most internal of the lateral abdominal muscles, the transverse abdominis muscle arises from the thoracolumbar fascia (lumbodorsal fascia), the iliac crest, the inguinal ligament, and the inner surfaces of the cartilages of the lower six ribs to run circumferentially and ventrally to terminate in the aponeurosis of the transversus abdominis muscle.

The transversus abdominis muscle is innervated by intercostal nerves T7 to T11, the subcostal nerve of T12, and the iliohypogastric and ilioinguinal branches of the first lumbar nerve.

Tonic abdominal muscle activation, at least in the upright posture, may serve an important "inspiratory" role. Abdominal muscle contraction and the movement of abdominal contents lengthen the diaphragm and increase its force (pressure) generating capabilities. This "inspiratory" action of abdominal muscles may be important for a variety of respiratory functions, including resting quiet breathing and speech production.

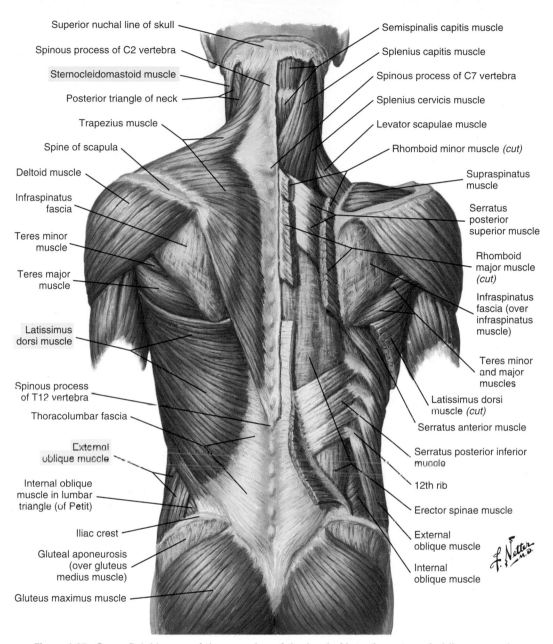

Superior nuchal line of skull

Spinous process of C2 vertebra

Sternocleidomastoid muscle

Posterior triangle of neck

Trapezius muscle

Spine of scapula

Deltoid muscle

Infraspinatus fascia

Teres minor muscle

Teres major muscle

Latissimus dorsi muscle

Spinous process of T12 vertebra

Thoracolumbar fascia

External oblique muscle

Internal oblique muscle in lumbar triangle (of Petit)

Iliac crest

Gluteal aponeurosis (over gluteus medius muscle)

Gluteus maximus muscle

Semispinalis capitis muscle

Splenius capitis muscle

Spinous process of C7 vertebra

Splenius cervicis muscle

Levator scapulae muscle

Rhomboid minor muscle (cut)

Supraspinatus muscle

Serratus posterior superior muscle

Rhomboid major muscle (cut)

Infraspinatus fascia (over infraspinatus muscle)

Teres minor and major muscles

Latissimus dorsi muscle (cut)

Serratus anterior muscle

Serratus posterior inferior muscle

12th rib

Erector spinae muscle

External oblique muscle

Internal oblique muscle

Figure 1.25. Superficial layers of the muscles of the back. Note the external oblique muscle.

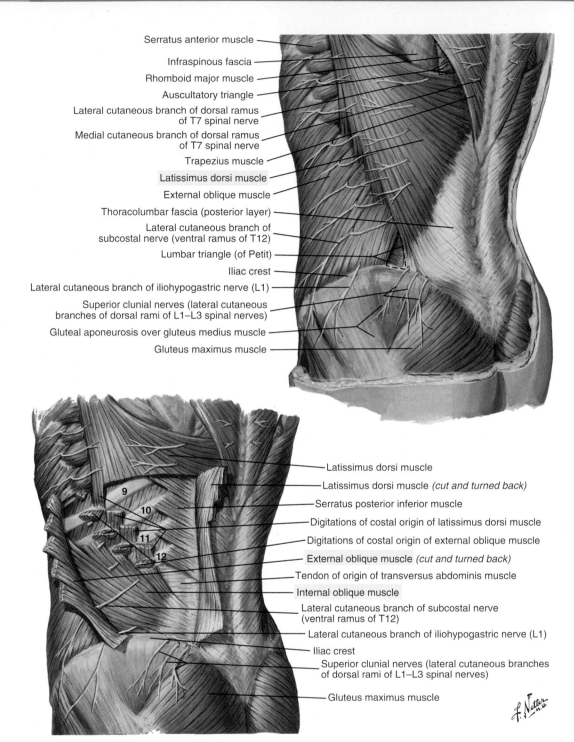

Serratus anterior muscle

Infraspinous fascia

Rhomboid major muscle

Auscultatory triangle

Lateral cutaneous branch of dorsal ramus
of T7 spinal nerve

Medial cutaneous branch of dorsal ramus
of T7 spinal nerve

Trapezius muscle

Latissimus dorsi muscle

External oblique muscle

Thoracolumbar fascia (posterior layer)

Lateral cutaneous branch of
subcostal nerve (ventral ramus of T12)

Lumbar triangle (of Petit)

Iliac crest

Lateral cutaneous branch of iliohypogastric nerve (L1)

Superior clunial nerves (lateral cutaneous
branches of dorsal rami of L1–L3 spinal nerves)

Gluteal aponeurosis over gluteus medius muscle

Gluteus maximus muscle

Latissimus dorsi muscle

Latissimus dorsi muscle (cut and turned back)

Serratus posterior inferior muscle

Digitations of costal origin of latissimus dorsi muscle

Digitations of costal origin of external oblique muscle

External oblique muscle (cut and turned back)

Tendon of origin of transversus abdominis muscle

Internal oblique muscle

Lateral cutaneous branch of subcostal nerve
(ventral ramus of T12)

Lateral cutaneous branch of iliohypogastric nerve (L1)

Iliac crest

Superior clunial nerves (lateral cutaneous branches
of dorsal rami of L1–L3 spinal nerves)

Gluteus maximus muscle

Figure 1.26. The posterolateral abdominal wall. Note the internal oblique muscle.

Principal Muscles of Inspiration

Muscle(s)	Origin	Insertion	Action(s)	Innervation
Diaphragm (see Figures 1.15 [p. 51] and 1.16 [p. 52]) **Three parts** 1. Sternal portion 2. Costal portion 3. Lumbar portion **Central tendon** Aponeurosis in which the three muscular parts insert **Openings** 1. The aorta passes behind the median arcuate ligament of the diaphragm (see Figure 1.16 [p. 52]) 2. Esophageal hiatus 3. Foramen of the inferior vena cava (caval opening)	1. Xiphoid process, inner surface 2. Costal cartilages and adjacent portions of the lower six ribs, inner surface 3. Superior lumbar vertebrae and medial and lateral arcuate ligaments	All insert into the central tendon	Contraction; pulls central tendon downward, increasing the vertical and anterolateral dimensions of the thorax	Phrenic nerves originating from cervical spinal nerves C3-C5
External intercostals (see Figure 1.21 [p. 59])	Inferior surface of the superior rib	Superior surface of the rib below	Expand the rib cage Stiffen the chest wall	Intercostal nerves (T1-T11)
Interchondral (parasternal) portion of internal intercostals (see Figure 1.22 [p. 61])	Inferior surface of rib spaces from the costochondral junction to the sternum	Superior surface of the rib below	Expand the rib cage Stiffen the chest wall	Intercostal nerves (T1-T11)

Accessory Muscles of Inspiration

Muscle(s)	Origin	Insertion	Action(s)	Innervation
Pectoralis major (see Figure 1.19 [p. 56])	Greater tubercle of the humerus	Clavicle Sternum Cartilages of ribs 1 or 2 through 6 or 7 Aponeurosis of external oblique	With arm fixed, portions of the muscle pull sternum and ribs upward during forced inspiration May also facilitate forced expiration by drawing the arms medially to compress the rib cage	Lateral and medial pectoral nerves (C5-C8 and T1)
Pectoralis minor (see Figure 1.21 [p. 59])	Coracoid process of the scapula	Outer surfaces of ribs 3-5	With the scapula fixed, elevates ribs 3-5 during forced inspiration	Lateral and medial pectoral nerves (C5-C8 and T1)
Serratus anterior (see Figure 1.19 [p. 56])	Inner, medial border of the scapula	Eight or nine upper ribs	With the scapula fixed, elevates upper ribs in forced inspiration	Long thoracic nerve (C5-C7)
Sternocleidomastoid (Figure 1.27; see also Figure 1.19 [p. 56])	Mastoid process of temporal bone	Sternum (manubrium) and clavicle	Raises the sternum and thus the ribs in forced inspiration	Spinal accessory nerve (cranial nerve XI) and cervical spinal nerves C2-C4
Quadratus lumborum (see Figures 1.16 [p. 52] and 1.18 [p. 55])	Iliolumbar ligament and posterior portion of the iliac crest	Medial half of the twelfth ribs and transverse processes of the superior lumbar vertebrae	Fixes the lower rib and provides a base for inspiratory movements of the diaphragm May aid in the precise relaxation of the diaphragm during the expiratory phases of speech and singing	Thoracic spinal nerve (T12) and lumbar spinal nerves (L1-L4)
Scalene muscles[a]: anterior, middle, and posterior (see Figure 1.27)	Transverse processes of cervical vertebrae C2-C7	Upper surfaces of first and second ribs	Elevate the ribs	Anterior: cervical spinal nerves C4-C6 Middle: C3-C8 Posterior: C6-C8

[a]Often listed as accessory muscles of respiration, scalene muscles have been shown to be consistently active during resting inspiration in a variety of animal species, including humans. Some authors therefore consider them to be principal muscles of inspiration.

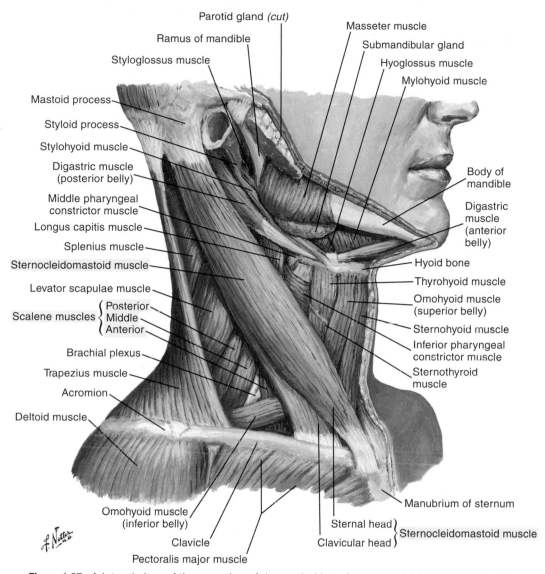

Figure 1.27. A lateral view of the muscles of the neck. Note the sternocleidomastoid muscle.

Principal Muscles of Expiration

Muscle(s)	Origin	Insertion	Action(s)	Innervation
Interosseous portion of internal intercostals (see Figure 1.24 [p. 63])	Inner superior surface of the rib below	Inner inferior surface of the rib above	Pull ribs downward Stiffen the chest wall	Intercostal nerves (T1-T11)
Rectus abdominis (Figures 1.28 and 1.29 [p. 72]; see also Figures 1.19 [p. 56] and 1.22 [p. 61])	Pubic symphysis and pubic crest	Costal cartilages of ribs 5-7 and xiphoid process of the sternum	Compresses abdomen	Intercostal nerves (T7-T11) Subcostal nerve (T12)
External oblique (see Figures 1.28 and 1.29 [p. 72]; see also Figures 1.19 [p. 56] and 1.23 [p. 62])	External surfaces of the eight lowest ribs	Iliac crest Inguinal ligament Aponeurosis of the external oblique	Compresses abdomen	Intercostal nerves (T7-T11) Subcostal nerve (T12)
Internal oblique (see Figures 1.28 and 1.29 [p. 72]; see also Figures 1.19 [p. 56] and 1.23 [p. 62])	Iliac crest Inguinal ligaments Thoracolumbar fascia	Costal cartilages of the lowest three or four ribs Aponeurosis of the internal oblique	Compresses abdomen	Intercostal nerves (T7-T11) Subcostal nerve (T12) First lumbar spinal nerve, L1 (iliohypogastric and ilioinguinal branches)
Transversus abdominis (Figures 1.29 [p. 72] and 1.30 [p. 73]; see also Figures 1.18 [p. 55], 1.21 [p. 59], and 1.23 [p. 62])	Iliac crest Inguinal ligaments Thoracolumbar fascia Inner surface of cartilages of the lower six ribs	Aponeurosis of the transversus abdominis	Compresses the abdomen	Intercostal nerves (T7-T11) Subcostal nerve (T12) First lumbar spinal nerve, L1 (iliohypogastric and ilioinguinal branches)
Transverse thoracis (triangularis sterni) (see Figure 1.24 [p. 63])	Internal surface of the rib cage from the sternum and costal cartilages 5-7	Internal surface of costal cartilages and adjacent portions of ribs 2-6	May pull the ribs slightly downward	Intercostal nerves (T2-T6)
Latissimus dorsi (see Figures 1.25 [p. 65] and 1.26 [p. 66])	Spinous process of the lower six thoracic vertebrae Thoracolumbar fascia Iliac crest Lower three or four ribs	Anterosuperior surface of the humerus	Compresses the thorax for forced expiration, such as for coughing With humerus fixed, also elevates ribs for forced inspiration	Thoracodorsal nerve (C6-C8)

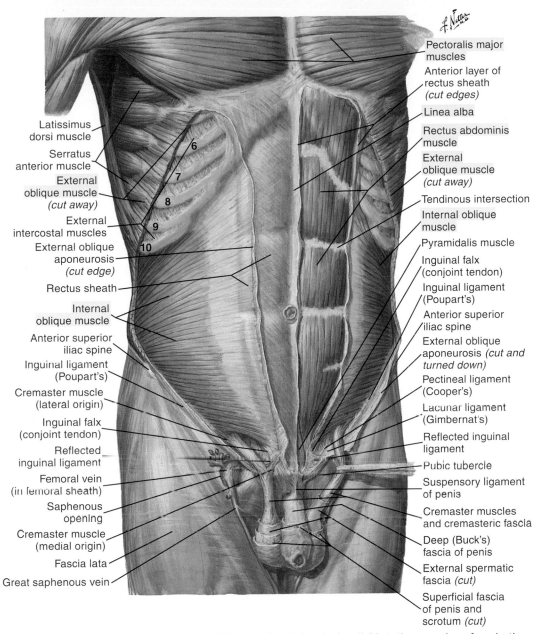

Pectoralis major muscles

Anterior layer of rectus sheath *(cut edges)*

Linea alba

Rectus abdominis muscle

External oblique muscle *(cut away)*

Tendinous intersection

Internal oblique muscle

Pyramidalis muscle

Inguinal falx (conjoint tendon)

Inguinal ligament (Poupart's)

Anterior superior iliac spine

External oblique aponeurosis *(cut and turned down)*

Pectineal ligament (Cooper's)

Lacunar ligament (Gimbernat's)

Reflected inguinal ligament

Pubic tubercle

Suspensory ligament of penis

Cremaster muscles and cremasteric fascia

Deep (Buck's) fascia of penis

External spermatic fascia *(cut)*

Superficial fascia of penis and scrotum *(cut)*

Latissimus dorsi muscle

Serratus anterior muscle

External oblique muscle *(cut away)*

External intercostal muscles

External oblique aponeurosis *(cut edge)*

Rectus sheath

Internal oblique muscle

Anterior superior iliac spine

Inguinal ligament (Poupart's)

Cremaster muscle (lateral origin)

Inguinal falx (conjoint tendon)

Reflected inguinal ligament

Femoral vein (in femoral sheath)

Saphenous opening

Cremaster muscle (medial origin)

Fascia lata

Great saphenous vein

6
7
8
9
10

Figure 1.28. An intermediate dissection of the anterior abdominal wall. Note the muscles of expiration.

Section above arcuate line

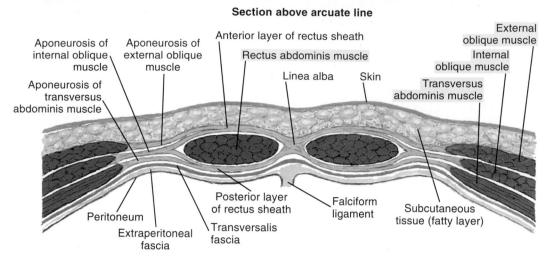

Aponeurosis of internal oblique muscle splits to form anterior and posterior layers of rectus sheath. Aponeurosis of external oblique muscle joins anterior layer of sheath; aponeurosis of transversus abdominis muscle joins posterior layer. Anterior and posterior layers of rectus sheath unite medially to form linea alba.

Section below arcuate line

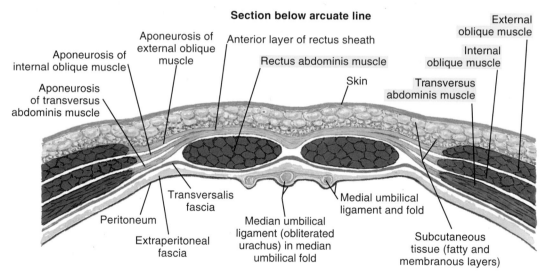

Aponeurosis of internal oblique muscle does not split at this level but passes completely anterior to rectus abdominis muscle and is fused there with both aponeurosis of external oblique muscle and that of transversus abdominis muscle. Thus, posterior wall of rectus sheath is absent below arcuate line, and rectus abdominis muscle lies on transversalis fascia.

Figure 1.29. Cross-sections of the rectus sheath. Note the aponeuroses of the external oblique, internal oblique, and transversus abdominis muscles.

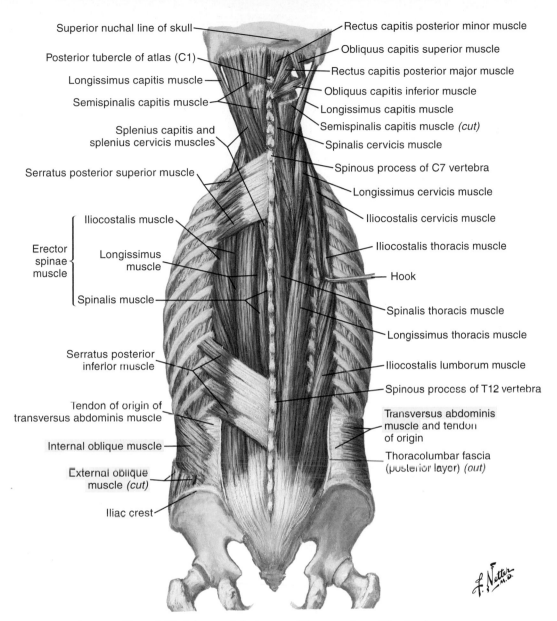

Superior nuchal line of skull
Posterior tubercle of atlas (C1)
Longissimus capitis muscle
Semispinalis capitis muscle
Splenius capitis and splenius cervicis muscles
Serratus posterior superior muscle

Erector spinae muscle
  Iliocostalis muscle
  Longissimus muscle
  Spinalis muscle

Serratus posterior inferior muscle
Tendon of origin of transversus abdominis muscle
Internal oblique muscle
External oblique muscle (cut)
Iliac crest

Rectus capitis posterior minor muscle
Obliquus capitis superior muscle
Rectus capitis posterior major muscle
Obliquus capitis inferior muscle
Longissimus capitis muscle
Semispinalis capitis muscle (cut)
Spinalis cervicis muscle
Spinous process of C7 vertebra
Longissimus cervicis muscle
Iliocostalis cervicis muscle
Iliocostalis thoracis muscle
Hook
Spinalis thoracis muscle
Longissimus thoracis muscle
Iliocostalis lumborum muscle
Spinous process of T12 vertebra
Transversus abdominis muscle and tendon of origin
Thoracolumbar fascia (posterior layer) (out)

Figure 1.30. Intermediate layers of the muscles of the back.

■ RESPIRATORY VOLUMES AND CAPACITIES

Volumes (Figure 1.31)

The different respiratory volumes are mutually exclusive, meaning that they do not overlap, and are as follows:

- **Tidal** volume is the volume (or amount) of air inspired or expired during normal, quiet breathing.
- **Inspiratory reserve** volume is the maximal amount of air that can be inspired above normal inspiratory tidal volume.
- **Expiratory reserve** volume is the maximal amount of air that can be expired below normal expiratory tidal volume.
- **Residual** volume is the amount of air remaining in the lungs after a maximal forced expiration (thus the lungs cannot be completely emptied voluntarily).

Capacities

Respiratory capacities are sums of volumes and are measured during the following pulmonary function tests:

- **Inspiratory** capacity is the total amount of air that can be inspired after a tidal expiration (tidal volume + inspiratory reserve volume).
- **Functional residual** capacity is the amount of air remaining in the lungs after a normal tidal expiration (expiratory reserve volume + residual volume).
- **Vital** capacity is the total amount of air that can be forcibly expired after a maximal inspiration (inspiratory reserve volume + tidal volume + expiratory reserve volume).
- **Total lung** capacity is the total amount of air after a maximal inspiration. It is the sum of all volumes (residual volume + expiratory reserve volume + tidal volume + inspiratory reserve volume).

Other Functional Measures

Minute ventilation is the amount of air moved into or out of the lungs per minute and is calculated by multiplying tidal volume by breaths per minute (respiratory rate).

   Physiological dead space is the volume of air remaining in the conducting airways (such as the bronchi, trachea, pharynx, and so on) that does not reach the alveoli and participate in gas exchange (referred to as *anatomical dead space*) and the volume of air that reaches the alveoli but does not exchange carbon dioxide or oxygen (referred to as *alveolar dead space*). Physiological dead space is nearly equal to anatomical dead space in healthy individuals.

   Alveolar ventilation is the volume of air per minute that reaches the alveoli *and* takes part in gas exchange. It is calculated by subtracting physiological dead space volume from tidal volume and multiplying by respiratory rate.

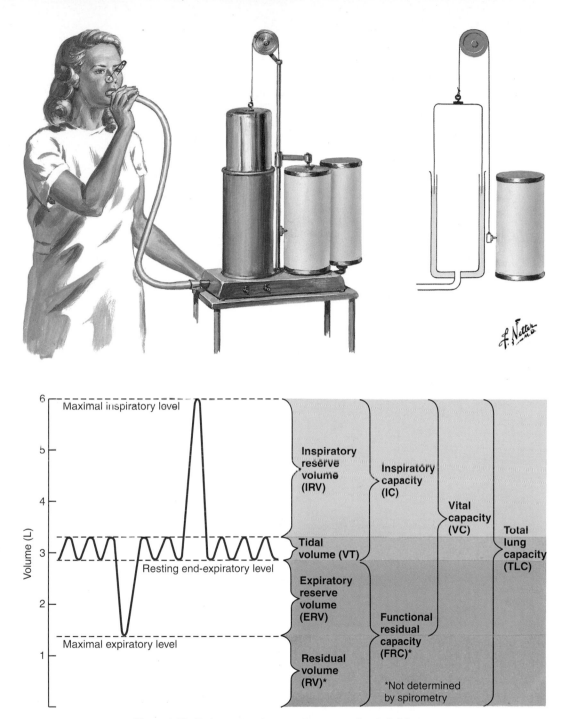

Figure 1.31. Spirometry: Lung volumes and subdivisions.

LARYNGEAL-PHONATORY SYSTEM

■ OVERVIEW

The larynx is formed of cartilages, membranes, and ligaments. It contains the vocal folds that function as a valve. The valve is opened (vocal fold abduction) or closed (adduction) through laryngeal muscle activation.

The larynx and vocal folds have three primary biological functions: (1) to protect the airway (e.g., during swallowing), (2) to trap air in the lungs in order to stabilize the torso during physical exertion, and (3) to modify upper airway resistance during quiet breathing to ensure adequate gas exchange. The vocal folds are slightly less abducted during the expiratory phase of the breathing cycle and work in concert with postinspiratory contraction of the diaphragm to ensure appropriate expiratory phase duration.

In addition to these primary biological functions, the larynx acts as an articulator, rapidly adducting and abducting the vocal folds, which are necessary for voiced (those that involve vocal fold vibration) and unvoiced sounds, respectively. This activity must be precisely timed with respiratory drive and supralaryngeal articulatory movements for specific sound production.

Vocal fold vibration begins when expiratory drive generates sufficient subglottal pressure to overcome the resistance of the adducted vocal folds and vocal folds open to release a burst of compressed air into the supraglottal space known as the *vocal tract*. The elasticity of the vocal folds and a Bernoulli effect act to close the vocal folds. The cycle repeats itself when subglottal pressure again overcomes the resistance of the vocal folds. Although much attention is given to the opening and closing of the vocal folds and to the fundamental frequency of the voice, vocal fold vibration generates a complex sound source that contains a fundamental frequency and harmonics. This complex sound source is modified by the resonant modes of the vocal tract to produce specific sounds such as vowels.

Variations in fundamental frequency (the rate of opening and closing of the vibrating vocal folds) and its perceptual correlate (pitch) serve important roles in speech production. Changes in fundamental frequency result from changes in the length and tension of the vocal folds, which in turn result from a complex interaction between intrinsic and extrinsic laryngeal muscles, with the cricothyroid playing crucial roles.

Increases in vocal intensity (loudness) are related to increases in subglottal pressure produced by increased expiratory drive against greater medial compression of the adducted vocal folds. Larger bursts of compressed air are released into the vocal tract, providing a sound source with greater acoustical energy.

Vocal fold closure and anterior and superior displacement of the hyoid bone and of the larynx (often referred to as "laryngeal elevation") are key contributors to airway protection during swallowing. High expiratory drive against adducted vocal folds is also a key component of cough, protecting the airway against the penetration and aspiration of foods and liquids.

The structures and muscles of the laryngeal-phonatory system are provided next.

■ LARYNX (Figures 2.1 and 2.2 [p. 83])

The larynx is approximately 5 cm in length and extends from the level of the third or fourth cervical vertebra to the sixth. It is located in the anterior portion of the neck, in front of the pharynx, above the trachea, and below the hyoid bone. The larynx functions as a two-way valve for the respiratory airway. It can function in this way because of two mobile muscular (and other soft tissue) bands called the *vocal folds*.

The structural framework of the larynx is composed of several paired and unpaired laryngeal cartilages and associated membranes and ligaments, as follows:

- Larger unpaired cartilages:
  - Thyroid cartilage
  - Cricoid cartilage
  - Epiglottis
- Smaller paired cartilages:
  - Arytenoid cartilages
  - Corniculate, or Santorini's, cartilages
  - Cuneiform cartilages
  - Triticeal cartilages

The epiglottis and the corniculate, cuneiform, and triticeal cartilages are formed of elastic cartilage; the rest are formed of hyaline cartilage, which may calcify with advancing age, with the exception of the arytenoid cartilages, which have a dense concentration of elastic cartilage in their vocal processes.

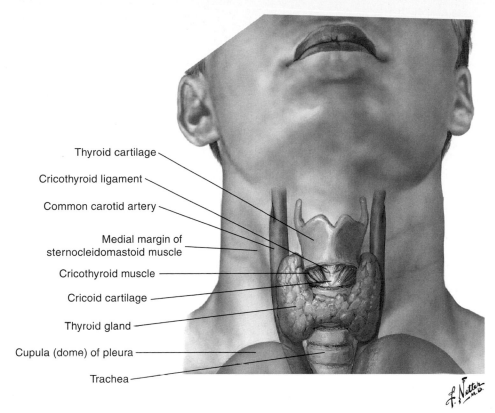

Thyroid cartilage

Cricothyroid ligament

Common carotid artery

Medial margin of
sternocleidomastoid muscle

Cricothyroid muscle

Cricoid cartilage

Thyroid gland

Cupula (dome) of pleura

Trachea

Figure 2.1. Position of the larynx, anterior view, In situ.

■ CARTILAGES OF THE LARYNX (Figure 2.2)

Thyroid Cartilage

Situated above and partially surrounding the cricoid cartilage, the thyroid cartilage is composed of two convex lateral, approximately quadrilateral laminae: the quadrilateral or thyroid laminae. These laminae fuse anteriorly to form the thyroid angle of approximately 120 degrees in adult females and 90 degrees in adult males. The more acute angle in the male (which develops during puberty) as contrasted to the female goes with longer and more massive vocal folds. This in turn relates to a lower fundamental frequency of vocal fold vibration (pitch) in adult males (approximately 125 Hz) versus females (approximately 210 Hz) because frequency is inversely proportional to mass.

- A palpable depression, or "notch," on the superior surface of the two fused laminae is called the *thyroid notch*. This notch lies directly superior to the laryngeal prominence, or "Adam's apple," which is more prominent (and visible) in males versus females. Horizontally, the notch lies approximately 6 to 9 mm above the vocal folds.
- There are two pairs of horns: two superior horns that articulate with the hyoid bone via the lateral thyrohyoid ligament (lateral thickening of the thyrohyoid membrane) and two smaller inferior horns that articulate with the cricoid cartilage.
- The oblique line on the lateral surface is the point of attachment of the sternothyroid, thyrohyoid, and thyropharyngeus (part of the inferior pharyngeal constrictor) muscles.
- The median (anterior) cricothyroid ligament attaches the thyroid with the cricoid anteriorly.

Cricoid Cartilage

Cricoid cartilage is situated just above the superior tracheal cartilage. It forms the inferior portion of the larynx and attaches to the trachea via the cricotracheal membrane or ligament. Cricoid cartilage forms a complete "signet" ring, as follows:

- The front is composed of a low anterior arch.
- The back is composed of a taller posterior quadrate (cricoid) lamina.
- The two paired points of articulation with synovial joints are as follows:
  - One point for the arytenoid cartilages is located on the superior surface of the quadrate lamina and allows for adduction and abduction of the paired vocal folds.
  - One point for the inferior horns of the thyroid cartilage is located on the lateral surface and allows for movement between the cricoid and thyroid cartilages to adjust the length and tension of the vocal folds.

Arytenoid Cartilages

The arytenoid cartilages are small pyramidal cartilages with the inferior concave surface, or base, resting on the convex arytenoid facets on the lateral border of the superior surface of the posterior quadrate lamina of the cricoid. The location and movement of these two cartilages are crucial to laryngeal function.

Three processes of the arytenoid cartilages are as follows:
1. The apex (the pyramid's summit) is the superior process.
2. The muscular process (site of muscular insertion) extends laterally.
3. The vocal process (site of vocal fold insertion) extends anteriorly.

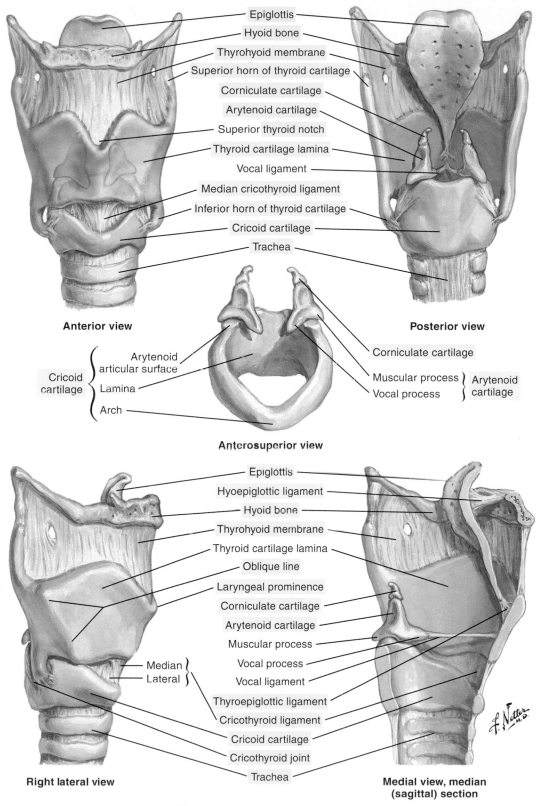

Figure 2.2. The laryngeal cartilages.

Note: Labels of certain figures are highlighted in yellow to emphasize the related elements in the corresponding text.

Corniculate, or Santorini's, Cartilages

Corniculate cartilages, or Santorini's cartilages, are elastic conical cartilages on the apex of the arytenoid cartilages.

Cuneiform Cartilages

Cuneiform cartilages (Figure 2.3 [p. 87]) are covered in soft tissue and situated within the aryepiglottic folds anterosuperior to the corniculate cartilages. Their presence is indicated by the cuneiform tubercles.

Triticeal (Tritiate) Cartilages

The triticeal cartilages are small cartilages located in the lateral hyothyroid ligaments (not present in all people).

Epiglottis

The epiglottis is a flexible elastic cartilage situated behind the median portion of the thyroid cartilage, which it exceeds superiorly. It is attached to the inner medial surface of the thyroid angle by the thyroepiglottic ligament. The epiglottis extends obliquely superiorly and posteriorly and attaches to the hyoid bone via the hyoepiglottic ligament. The aryepiglottic fold extends from the lateral margins of the epiglottis to the apexes of the arytenoids.

The epiglottis is attached to the root of the tongue via the median and lateral glossoepiglottic folds that create the valleculae (see Part 3: Oropharyngeal-Articulatory System, p. 119). The pyriform (piriform) sinus (fossa) are small lateral cavities between the aryepiglottic fold (medially) and the thyroid cartilage and thyrohyoid membrane (laterally) (see Part 3: Oropharyngeal-Articulatory System, p. 119). The "tipping" of the epiglottis during laryngeal elevation for swallowing may assist in protecting the lower airway.

■ HYOID BONE (see Figure 2.2 [p. 83])

The hyoid bone provides support for the tongue and the larynx, but it is not generally considered a part of the larynx. It is a "floating" bone that does not have direct contact with any other bone. It is instead attached by a complex system of muscles and ligaments from the tongue and the extrinsic muscles of the larynx and other facial, cranial, and skeletal structures. It is therefore a very mobile structure acted on by several muscle systems.

Located in the neck at the level of the third cervical vertebrae, it is oriented horizontally and has a horseshoe-like shape with the following components:
- A rectangular body (corpus)
- A pair of lesser horns (cornua)
- A pair of greater horns (cornua)

■ TYPES OF JOINTS (see Figure 2.2 [p. 83])

Three types of joints exist, each differing in its degree of mobility, as follows:
1. The fibrous joint is immobile.
2. The cartilaginous joint is slightly mobile.
3. The synovial joint is highly mobile.

The two important points of articulation and associated joints of the larynx are as follows:
- The cricothyroid is the synovial joint between the lesser horn (inferior horn) of the thyroid cartilage and the articular facets of the cricoid. This joint allows for two types of movements: (1) forward "bending" of the thyroid over the cricoid and (2) anteroposterior gliding of the thyroid in the horizontal axis. Each of these movements potentially affects the length (and tension) of the vocal folds.
- The cricoarytenoid is the synovial joint between the base of the arytenoids and the superior surface of the quadrate lamina of the cricoid. It allows the arytenoids to rock toward (inferiorly medially) or away from (superiorly laterally) the interior of the cricoid, bringing the vocal processes and, consequently, the vocal folds into adduction and abduction, respectively.

■ LIGAMENTS AND MEMBRANES

The laryngeal cartilages are linked together and to adjacent structures by extrinsic and intrinsic ligaments and membranes.

Extrinsic Ligaments and Membranes (see Figure 2.2 [p. 83])

The function of the extrinsic ligaments and membranes is to suspend and link the larynx to the following adjacent structures.

Thyrohyoid (Hyothyroid) Membrane and Ligaments

The thyrohyoid membrane lies between the superior border of the thyroid cartilage and the hyoid bone. It becomes thicker medially to form the median (middle) thyrohyoid ligament. This membrane also becomes thicker posteriorly and laterally to form the lateral thyrohyoid ligaments, which link the superior horns of the thyroid to the hyoid bone.

Hyoepiglottic Ligament

The hyoepiglottic ligament links the anterior surface of the epiglottis to the inner surface of the superior surface of the body of the hyoid.

Cricotracheal Membrane

The cricotracheal membrane joins the superior border of the first tracheal ring to the inferior surface of the cricoid.

Intrinsic Ligaments and Membranes (Figure 2.3)

The function of the intrinsic ligaments and membranes is to link and support the laryngeal cartilages. Most of the intrinsic laryngeal membranes arise from a sheet of connective tissue called the *fibroelastic membrane.* Its inferior division is called the *conus elasticus,* and the superior portion is called the *quadrangular membrane.*

Quadrangular Membrane

The quadrangular membrane is formed of paired membranes that extend from the lateral edge of the epiglottis and the angle of the thyroid cartilage. These extend posteriorly and inferiorly to the corniculate cartilages and the medial borders of the arytenoids. The quadrangular membrane is wider superiorly and narrows inferiorly to form the vestibular ligament.

The aryepiglottic folds form the superior border of the quadrangular membrane and extend from the lateral surface of the epiglottis to the apexes of the arytenoids. The cuneiform and corniculate cartilages are embedded in these folds.

Conus Elasticus, Cricovocal Membrane, or Lateral Cricothyroid Ligament or Membrane

The conus elasticus is a cone-shaped, thin, continuous membrane that extends from the superior surface of the cricoid cartilage to the median border of the vocal folds, where it terminates as the vocal ligaments. These ligaments extend from the vocal process of the arytenoid cartilages to the angle of the thyroid cartilage and form a portion of the vocal folds.

The conus elasticus is sometimes considered to include the median cricothyroid ligament (see Figure 2.2 [p. 83]), which is a well-defined elastic tissue that extends from the superior surface of the cricoid arch to the inferior border of the thyroid cartilage near the angle of the thyroid.

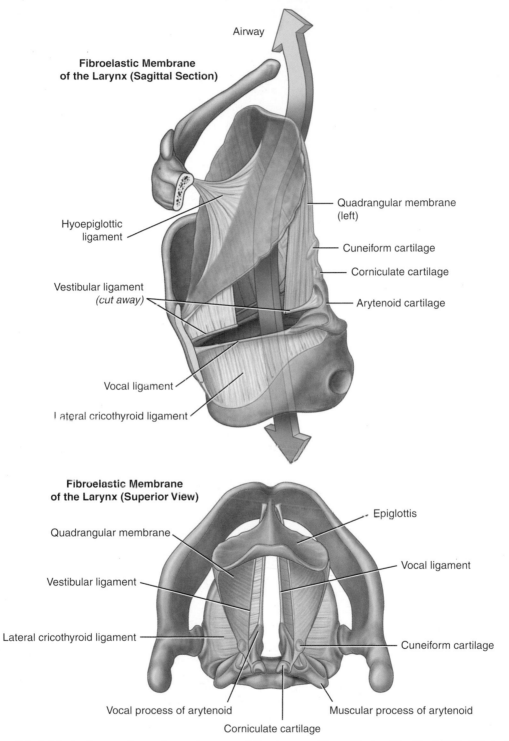

Figure 2.3. Intrinsic ligaments and membranes of the larynx. (From Drake RL, Vogl AW, Mitchell AWM: *Gray's anatomy for students,* ed 3, Philadelphia, 2015, Churchill Livingstone.)

■ VOCAL FOLDS (Figures 2.4, 2.5 [p. 90], and 2.6 [p. 91])

Throughout this atlas, the term *vocal folds* is used to designate the structures involved in the generation of the laryngeal sound source of speech. Although the term *vocal cords* is perhaps better known to the general public, the term *vocal folds* is the more appropriate anatomical term to designate these key laryngeal structures.

The use of the term *vocal cords* comes from the early anatomical inspections of the larynx, when these structures appeared as "cords" because of the appearance of the thickened vocal ligaments (see Figure 2.5 [p. 90]). Since then, our understanding of the complex structure and function of the vibration of the vocal folds has advanced. We know that simple "cords" obviously cannot prevent foreign objects from entering the lower airway, but vocal folds acting as a valve can. There are actually two pairs of vocal folds arranged in parallel and in an anteroposterior orientation, which can be most clearly seen in a coronal section of the larynx (see Figure 2.6 [p. 91]) and described as the following:

- The false vocal folds (vestibular or ventricular folds) do not normally generate a sound source.
- The true vocal folds are inferior to the false vocal folds and are separated from the false vocal folds by a small fissure called the *laryngeal ventricle.*
- The laryngeal vestibule (supraglottic cavity) is superior to the false vocal folds.
- The infraglottic (subglottic) cavity extends from the inferior border of the true folds to the inferior border of the cricoid cartilage.
- The glottic region, which is also known as the *glottis,* corresponds to the space between the true vocal folds.
- The aryepiglottic folds form the "collar" or point of constriction of the entryway to the larynx (laryngeal inlet).
- The quadrangular membrane is located above the true vocal folds.
- The conus elasticus is the membranous covering in the subglottic region.

The vocal folds extend from the vocal process of the arytenoids to the inner surface of the thyroid cartilage. More precisely, they meet at the midline of the thyroid angle, between the thyroid notch and the inferior border of the thyroid cartilage.

Although estimates vary, vocal fold lengths generally have the following ranges:

- Men: 17 to 25 mm
- Women: 13 to 18 mm

The thickness of the vocal folds is approximately 5 mm.

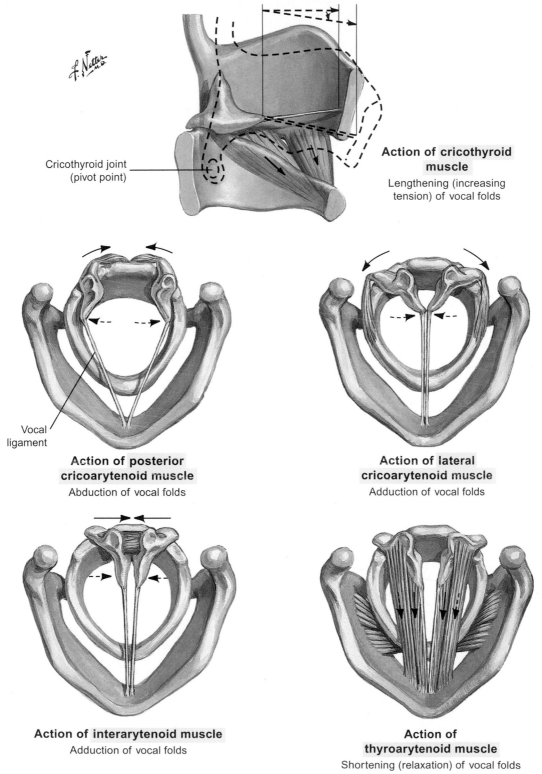

Cricothyroid joint
(pivot point)

Action of cricothyroid muscle
Lengthening (increasing tension) of vocal folds

Vocal ligament

Action of posterior cricoarytenoid muscle
Abduction of vocal folds

Action of lateral cricoarytenoid muscle
Adduction of vocal folds

Action of interarytenoid muscle
Adduction of vocal folds

Action of thyroarytenoid muscle
Shortening (relaxation) of vocal folds

Figure 2.4. Actions of the intrinsic muscles of the larynx. Solid arrows indicate the direction of muscle contraction. Dotted arrows indicate the resulting action of the muscular contraction on the laryngeal cartilages and, consequently, on the vocal folds.

Laryngoscopic View of the Larynx: Inspiration

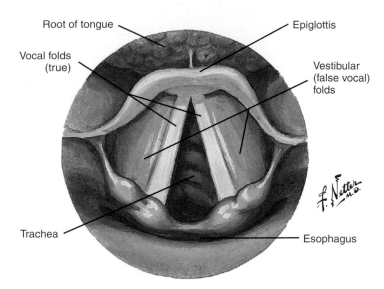

Figure 2.5. Abduction of the vocal folds during inspiration.

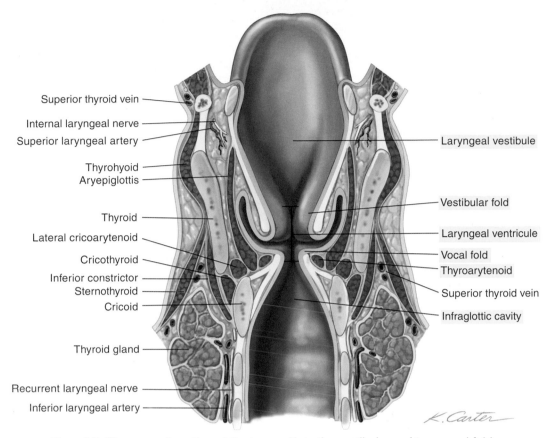

Figure 2.6. The coronal section of the larynx. Note the vestibular and true vocal folds.

Tissue Layers of the Vocal Folds

The vocal folds of an adult are composed of five layers of tissue: (1) the epithelium, (2) the superficial layer, (3) the intermediate layer, (4) the deep layer, and (5) the thyroarytenoid muscle. Each layer differs in terms of thickness and rigidity.

Epithelium

The epithelium is stratified, has a thickness of approximately 0.05 to 0.10 mm, and is the rigid layer that maintains the shape of the vocal folds. Under the epithelium is a composite structure of three layers called the *lamina propria*. The lamina propria has a thickness of 1 mm. The epithelium is attached to the superficial layer of the lamina propria by a complex basement membrane.

Superficial Layer (Reinke's Space)

The superficial layer, or Reinke's space, is composed of loosely organized fibers that form a gelatinous-like matrix approximately 0.5 mm thick. This layer is responsible for much of the vibratory movements of the vocal folds.

Intermediate Layer

The intermediate layer is formed by elastic fibers and in cross-section appears to resemble a bunch of cut, supple rubber bands.

Deep Layer

The deep layer is formed primarily by collagen fibers, with the consistency of a group of large cotton threads. The intermediate and deep layers form the vocal ligament and together are approximately 1 to 2 mm thick.

Thyroarytenoid Muscle

The thyroarytenoid muscle forms the bulk of the vocal folds, and its muscular fibers have the consistency of a packet of rigid rubber bands.

Classifications of Vocal Fold Layers

A variety of biomechanical models have been proposed to explain the vibratory or oscillatory behavior of the vocal folds during phonation. Within a biomechanical perspective, the vocal folds can be grouped into the following functional divisions:

- The cover consists of the epithelium (mucosa) and the superficial layer of the lamina propria (layers 1 and 2).
- The transition consists of the intermediate and deep layers of the lamina propria (layers 3 and 4), which together form the vocal ligament.
- The body consists of the thyroarytenoid muscle (layer 5).

Another two-layer biomechanical scheme combines layers 1 through 3 to form the cover and layers 4 and 5 to form the body.

From a simplified biomechanical perspective, changes in the length, rigidity (tension), and mass of the vocal folds determine the fundamental frequency of vocal fold vibration and its perceptual correlate of pitch. These parameters, and thus fundamental frequency, are thought to be regulated primarily through activation of the cricothyroid and thyroarytenoid muscles, with the cricothyroid muscle being the primary controller.

The cricothyroid muscle controls fundamental frequency by lengthening and thinning the vocal folds, which increases longitudinal tension and results in increased fundamental frequency.

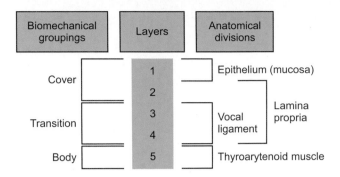

The contribution of the thyroarytenoid muscle is potentially more complex and may act by raising or lowering the fundamental frequency depending upon the degree of cricothyroid co-activation and the frequency range being produced (such as high or low pitch).

Blood Supply

The superior laryngeal branch (superior laryngeal artery) of the superior thyroid artery (a branch of the external carotid artery) supplies the superior part of the larynx. The inferior laryngeal branch of the inferior thyroid artery (from the thyrocervical trunk) supplies the inferior part of the larynx.

Innervation

The laryngeal muscles and their associated structures are innervated by the following two branches of the vagus nerve[1] (cranial nerve X):
1. The internal branch of the superior laryngeal nerve provides sensory innervation for the mucous membrane of the larynx above the vocal folds. The external branch provides motor innervation for the cricothyroid muscle.
2. The recurrent laryngeal nerve provides motor innervation of all intrinsic laryngeal muscles, except for the cricothyroid muscle. It has a sensory function for the mucous membranes below the vocal folds.

A third branch, the pharyngeal nerve, innervates primarily the muscles and mucous membranes of the pharynx and soft palate with the contribution of the glossopharyngeal (cranial nerve IX) and trigeminal (cranial nerve V) nerves.

The term *recurrent* means "returns, goes back to its origin." The recurrent laryngeal nerves distribute widely (particularly on the left side) before returning to provide motor innervation to laryngeal muscles. In their trajectory, the recurrent laryngeal nerves pass near many structures that make them vulnerable to disease and damage during surgical intervention.

---

[1]The name of the vagus nerve comes from the word *vagabond,* which is related to its large distribution.

■ MUSCLES OF THE LARYNX

The following two types of muscles affect laryngeal function:

1. The intrinsic muscles, which have their points of attachment within the skeletal framework of the larynx
2. The extrinsic muscles, which have one point of attachment on the laryngeal structures and another attachment outside of the larynx

These muscles will be discussed by stressing their impact on the vibratory characteristics of the vocal folds for phonation.

Intrinsic Muscles of the Larynx (Figure 2.7)

The intrinsic muscles of the larynx have their origin and insertion within the larynx. Five intrinsic muscles control the following:

• Adduction-abduction
• Tension-relaxation of the vocal folds

For adduction, the vocal processes (and the attached vocal folds) are rotated medially and inferiorly; for abduction, the vocal processes are rotated superiorly and laterally.

During phonation, the following two types of adjustments are made:

1. Variation of the medial compression or the degree of force by which the vocal folds are joined at the median line
2. Variation of the longitudinal tension or the degree of stretching of the vocal folds

Thyroarytenoid Muscle

The thyroarytenoid muscle forms the major mass of the vocal folds and, consequently, the major portion of the laryngeal "valve" that protects the airway and serves other primary biological functions, as previously mentioned. Its anterior origin is the inner surface of the thyroid, below the notch and near the thyroid angle. Taken as a whole, this muscle courses posteriorly to insert on the arytenoid cartilage, from the vocal to the muscular processes. It is deep to, and bounded medially by, the vocal ligament. The thyroarytenoid muscle is often divided into two functional parts or two subdivisions:

1. Thyrovocalis: medial portion (the vocalis or internal thyroarytenoid)
2. Thyromuscularis: lateral portion (muscularis or external thyroarytenoid)

Isolated, unopposed contraction of the thyroarytenoid shortens and thickens the body of the vocal folds, but loosens its cover. The impact on fundamental frequency of vibration of the vocal folds depends upon the degree of co-contraction of the cricothyroid and the frequency range being produced. Muscle shortening and increased mass may contribute to vocal fold adduction.

The thyroarytenoid muscle is innervated by the anterior division (also known as the *inferior laryngeal nerve*) of the recurrent laryngeal nerve.

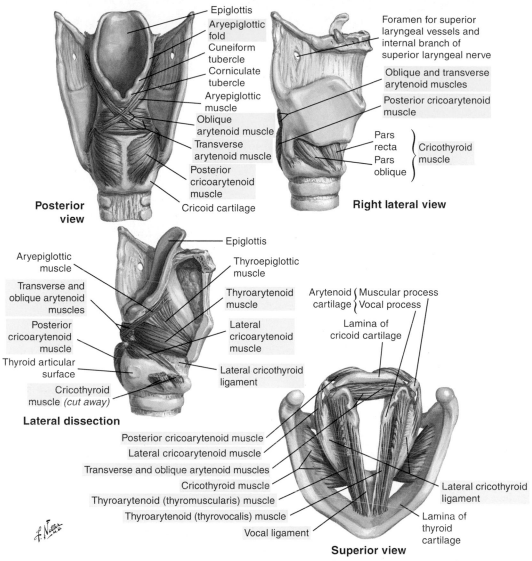

Posterior view

- Epiglottis
- Aryepiglottic fold
- Cuneiform tubercle
- Corniculate tubercle
- Aryepiglottic muscle
- Oblique arytenoid muscle
- Transverse arytenoid muscle
- Posterior cricoarytenoid muscle
- Cricoid cartilage

Right lateral view

- Foramen for superior laryngeal vessels and internal branch of superior laryngeal nerve
- Oblique and transverse arytenoid muscles
- Posterior cricoarytenoid muscle
- Pars recta / Pars oblique } Cricothyroid muscle

Lateral dissection

- Aryepiglottic muscle
- Transverse and oblique arytenoid muscles
- Posterior cricoarytenoid muscle
- Thyroid articular surface
- Cricothyroid muscle *(cut away)*
- Epiglottis
- Thyroepiglottic muscle
- Thyroarytenoid muscle
- Lateral cricoarytenoid muscle
- Lateral cricothyroid ligament

Superior view

- Arytenoid cartilage { Muscular process / Vocal process
- Lamina of cricoid cartilage
- Lateral cricothyroid ligament
- Lamina of thyroid cartilage

- Posterior cricoarytenoid muscle
- Lateral cricoarytenoid muscle
- Transverse and oblique arytenoid muscles
- Cricothyroid muscle
- Thyroarytenoid (thyromuscularis) muscle
- Thyroarytenoid (thyrovocalis) muscle
- Vocal ligament

Figure 2.7. The intrinsic muscles of the larynx.

Cricothyroid Muscle

The cricothyroid muscle is a major contributor to increasing vocal fold length and tension (vocal fold tensor) and may also assist in vocal fold abduction.

This muscle has the following two divisions:

1. The upper, more vertically directed portion (pars recta) courses from the anterior portion of the cricoid arch just lateral to the median line to the inferior surface of the thyroid cartilage.
2. The lower oblique portion (pars oblique) arises from the anterior portion of the cricoid arch (laterally to the median line) and courses posteriorly and superiorly to insert on the inferior border of the inferior horn of the thyroid cartilage.

The exact actions of the two portions of the cricothyroid are controversial. The pars recta is thought to rotate the thyroid cartilage inferiorly, and the pars oblique is thought to pull the thyroid anteriorly. This increases the distance between the thyroid and arytenoid cartilages, and because of the attachment of the vocal folds between these two cartilages, increases the length and tension of the vocal folds.

The cricothyroid muscle is innervated by the external branch of the superior laryngeal nerve.

Posterior Cricoarytenoid Muscle

The posterior cricoarytenoid muscle is a fan-shaped muscle and is the only abductor muscle of the vocal folds. It arises from the posterior quadrate lamina of the cricoid, and fibers course superiorly and laterally to insert onto the posterior surface of the muscular process of the arytenoid. This muscle is often divided into two parts, a medial belly and a lateral belly. Its action is to rotate the muscular processes downward and toward the midline, which moves the vocal processes laterally and superiorly, lengthening, elevating, and abducting the vocal folds (opens the glottis).

The posterior cricoarytenoid muscle is innervated by the posterior branch of the recurrent laryngeal nerve.

Lateral Cricoarytenoid Muscle

The lateral cricoarytenoid muscle is a vocal fold adductor. It arises from the superior surface of the lateral border of the cricoid arch, courses superiorly and posteriorly, and inserts on the anterior portion of the muscular process of the arytenoids. The contraction of the lateral cricoarytenoid muscle pulls on the muscular process and rotates the vocal processes toward the median line, which adducts the vocal folds (closes the glottis).

The lateral cricoarytenoid muscle is innervated by the anterior division of the recurrent laryngeal nerve.

Interarytenoid (Arytenoid) Muscle

The interarytenoid (arytenoid) muscle is also an adductor muscle, with the following two parts:
1. The transverse portion is the deeper portion, with horizontally directed fibers from the lateral margin of one arytenoid (between the muscular process and the apex) to the lateral margin of the other.
2. The oblique portion is more superficial, with obliquely directed fibers from the base of the muscular process of one arytenoid to the apex of the other. Some fibers continue superiorly to become the aryepiglottic muscle.

The action of the interarytenoid muscle is to pull the two arytenoids toward the midline and thus adduct the vocal folds. The muscle is also involved in the regulation of medial compression between the vocal folds.

The interarytenoid is innervated by the anterior division of the recurrent laryngeal nerve.

Extrinsic Muscles of the Larynx (Figures 2.8 and 2.9 [p. 101])

All of the extrinsic muscles have one point of attachment on a laryngeal structure or a structure that influences laryngeal position and movement (e.g., the hyoid bone). They contribute to the suspension, support, and mobility of the larynx. Extrinsic laryngeal muscles are further classified by whether they are located above or below the hyoid bone.

Actions of the extrinsic muscles are classified in the following two basic groups:

1. Four infrahyoid muscles are sometimes classified as laryngeal "depressors."
2. Four suprahyoid muscles are sometimes classified as laryngeal "elevators."

Infrahyoid Muscles

The isolated (unopposed) action of the four infrahyoid muscles is to move the larynx downward and to bring the thyroid cartilage closer to the hyoid bone. In collaboration with other muscles (suprahyoid muscles), the function of the infrahyoid muscles is to stabilize (fix) the hyoid bone to provide a firm base for jaw opening and for the movements of the tongue necessary for speech and swallowing.

Thyrohyoid Muscle

The thyrohyoid muscle is located deep to the superior portion of the sternohyoid muscle. It courses from the oblique line of the thyroid cartilage to the greater horn of the hyoid bone. Contraction of the thyrohyoid muscle approximates the thyroid cartilage and hyoid bone. Depending on which point of attachment is most mobile and the simultaneous activation of other muscles, the thyrohyoid muscle can pull down on the hyoid bone or lift the thyroid cartilage. Thus this muscle can be classified as either a laryngeal elevator or a laryngeal depressor. As a laryngeal elevator, it contributes to the opening of the pharyngoesophageal segment (upper esophageal sphincter) for swallowing.

Sternohyoid Muscle

The sternohyoid muscle courses from the sternum to the hyoid bone. It can pull down the hyoid bone and, with it, the larynx.

Omohyoid Muscle

The omohyoid muscle is a two-bellied muscle (inferior and superior) that extends from the scapula to the hyoid bone through an intermediate tendon. Contraction can pull down the hyoid bone.

Sternothyroid Muscle

The sternothyroid muscle is located deep to the sternohyoid muscle and courses from the sternum and first costal cartilage to the oblique line of the thyroid. Contraction of this muscle results in downward movement of the thyroid. It also may shorten the vocal folds, decreasing their tension and frequency of vibration.

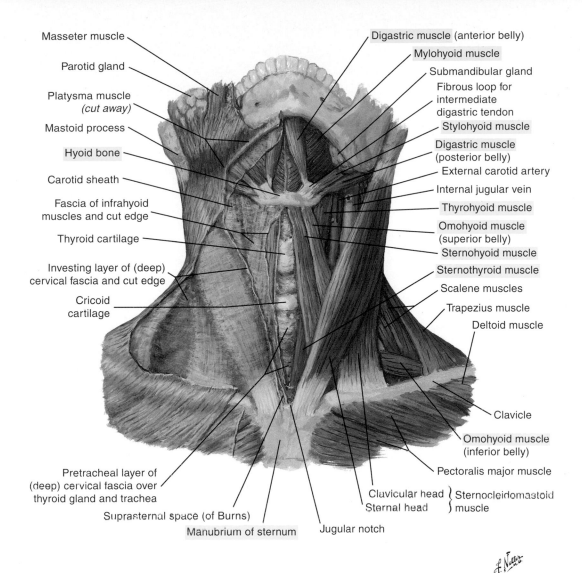

Masseter muscle

Parotid gland

Platysma muscle
(cut away)

Mastoid process

Hyoid bone

Carotid sheath

Fascia of infrahyoid
muscles and cut edge

Thyroid cartilage

Investing layer of (deep)
cervical fascia and cut edge

Cricoid
cartilage

Digastric muscle (anterior belly)

Mylohyoid muscle

Submandibular gland

Fibrous loop for
intermediate
digastric tendon

Stylohyoid muscle

Digastric muscle
(posterior belly)

External carotid artery

Internal jugular vein

Thyrohyoid muscle

Omohyoid muscle
(superior belly)

Sternohyoid muscle

Sternothyroid muscle

Scalene muscles

Trapezius muscle

Deltoid muscle

Clavicle

Omohyoid muscle
(inferior belly)

Pectoralis major muscle

Clavicular head } Sternocleidomastoid
Sternal head } muscle

Pretracheal layer of
(deep) cervical fascia over
thyroid gland and trachea

Suprasternal space (of Burns)

Manubrium of sternum

Jugular notch

Figure 2.8. An anterior view of the muscles of the neck. Note the four infrahyoid muscles:
(1) thyrohyoid, (2) sternohyoid, (3) omohyoid, and (4) sternothyroid.

Suprahyoid Muscles

When the hyoid is fixed by the infrahyoid muscles, suprahyoid muscle contraction opens the jaw by pulling down the mandible. Suprahyoid muscles can also elevate the hyoid bone and move the larynx upward, forward, or backward. During the act of swallowing, the activation of the suprahyoid muscles results in the anterior and superior displacement of the hyoid bone and of the larynx (often referred to as the "hyolaryngeal complex"), which facilitates the approximation of the arytenoid cartilage to the epiglottic base and the "tipping" of the epiglottis (as a result of biomechanical linkage). Together these mechanisms contribute to laryngeal vestibular closure as the bolus passes though the pharynx. The displacement of the hyoid bone and larynx also contributes to pharyngoesophageal segment (upper esophageal sphincter) opening, which allows the bolus to flow from the pharynx to the cervical esophagus.

The four muscles are as follows:

1. Digastric muscle
2. Mylohyoid muscle
3. Geniohyoid muscle
4. Stylohyoid muscle

These muscles all have a point of attachment on the skull or the mandible and another point of attachment on the hyoid bone. Because they play important roles in mastication, swallowing, and the articulatory movements of speech production, the mylohyoid, geniohyoid, and digastric muscles are examined in further detail in Part 3: Oropharyngeal-Articulatory System, pp. 148–149. The stylohyoid muscle is detailed in the table describing extrinsic muscles of the larynx on p. 104.

Cricopharyngeus Muscle

The cricopharyngeus muscle is part of the inferior constrictor muscle forming a portion of the pharynx. It plays an important role in swallowing (see Part 3: Oropharyngeal-Articulatory System, p. 155 and p. 160).

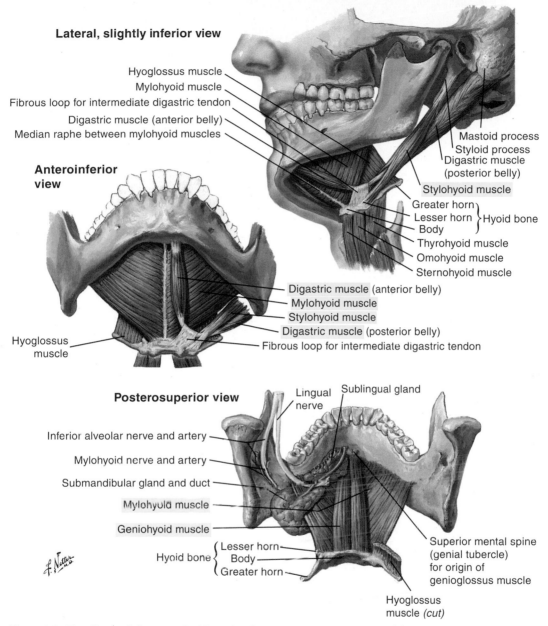

Lateral, slightly inferior view

Hyoglossus muscle
Mylohyoid muscle
Fibrous loop for intermediate digastric tendon
Digastric muscle (anterior belly)
Median raphe between mylohyoid muscles

Mastoid process
Styloid process
Digastric muscle (posterior belly)
Stylohyoid muscle
Greater horn
Lesser horn } Hyoid bone
Body
Thyrohyoid muscle
Omohyoid muscle
Sternohyoid muscle

Anteroinferior view

Digastric muscle (anterior belly)
Mylohyoid muscle
Stylohyoid muscle
Digastric muscle (posterior belly)
Fibrous loop for intermediate digastric tendon

Hyoglossus muscle

Posterosuperior view

Lingual nerve
Sublingual gland

Inferior alveolar nerve and artery
Mylohyoid nerve and artery
Submandibular gland and duct
Mylohyoid muscle
Geniohyoid muscle

Hyoid bone { Lesser horn
Body
Greater horn

Superior mental spine (genial tubercle) for origin of genioglossus muscle

Hyoglossus muscle (cut)

Figure 2.9. The floor of the mouth. Note the four suprahyoid muscles: (1) digastric, (2) mylohyoid, (3) geniohyoid, and (4) stylohyoid.

Intrinsic Muscles of the Larynx (see Figures 2.4 [p. 89] and 2.7 [p. 95])

Muscles	Description	Origin	Insertion	Action(s)	Innervation
Thyroarytenoid muscle, sometimes divided into two parts: thyromuscularis (muscularis) and thyrovocalis (vocalis) muscles	Muscle fibers contributing to the vocal folds	Inner surface of the thyroid	Vocal and muscular processes of the arytenoids	May increase or decrease fundamental frequency depending on the co-activation of other intrinsic muscles such as the cricothyroid	Recurrent laryngeal nerve of the vagus (cranial nerve X)
Cricothyroid	Fan-shaped muscle located between the cricoid and the thyroid cartilages, with two divisions: (1) pars recta and (2) pars oblique	Cricoid arch	Inferior border of the lamina and inferior horn of the thyroid	Decreases the distance between the thyroid and the cricoid Pulls thyroid anteriorly, lengthening and thinning the vocal folds and increasing longitudinal tension and pitch (tensor)	External branch of the superior laryngeal nerve of the vagus (cranial nerve X)
Posterior cricoarytenoid	Fan-shaped muscle on the posterior surface of the cricoid	Quadrate lamina of the cricoid	Posterior surface of the muscular process of the arytenoid	Laterally rotates the arytenoids and opens the glottis (abductor)	Recurrent laryngeal nerve of the vagus (cranial nerve X)
Lateral cricoarytenoid	Located deep to the thyroid cartilage	Superior surface of the anterolateral border of the cricoid arch	Anterior surface of the muscular process of the arytenoid	Medially rotates the arytenoids and closes the glottis (adductor)	Recurrent laryngeal nerve of the vagus (cranial nerve X)
Interarytenoid	Nonpaired muscle composed of fibers oriented in oblique and transverse direction; oblique fibers cross between the arytenoids to form an X and are located superficial to the transverse fibers	**Oblique fibers** Base of the muscular process of one arytenoid **Transverse fibers** Lateral border of the arytenoid, between the muscular process and the apex	**Oblique fibers** Apex of the opposite arytenoid Continuous with aryepiglottic muscle fibers **Transverse fibers** Lateral border of the opposite arytenoid	Approximates the arytenoids and closes the glottis (adductor)	Recurrent laryngeal nerve of the vagus (cranial nerve X)

Extrinsic Muscles of the Larynx (Infrahyoid Muscles) (Figure 2.10 [p. 105])

Muscles	Description	Origin	Insertion	Action(s)	Innervation
Thyrohyoid	Thin muscle that appears as a continuation of the sternohyoid muscle	Oblique line of the thyroid cartilage	Inferior border of the body and the greater horn of the hyoid bone	Approximates the hyoid and thyroid	First cervical spinal nerve (C1) traveling with fibers of the hypoglossal nerve (cranial nerve XII)
Sternohyoid	Thin muscle on the anterior surface of the neck	Posterior surface of the manubrium and medial border of the clavicle	Inferior border of the body of the hyoid bone	Depresses the hyoid	Cervical spinal nerves C1-C3 via ansa cervicalis
Omohyoid	Thin, narrow muscle, with superior and inferior bellies joined by a central tendon connected by deep fascia to the clavicle	Superior border of the scapula	Inferior border of the body of the hyoid	Depresses the hyoid	**Inferior belly** Cervical spinal nerves C1-C3 via ansa cervicalis **Posterior belly** First cervical spinal nerve (C1) via superior ramus of the ansa cervicalis
Sternothyroid	Long, thin muscle on the anterior surface of the neck	Posterior surface of the manubrium and first costal cartilage	Oblique line of the thyroid cartilage	Depresses the thyroid cartilage	Cervical spinal nerves C1-C3 via ansa cervicalis

Extrinsic Muscles of the Larynx (Suprahyoid Muscles) (Figure 2.11 [p. 106])

Muscles	Description	Origin	Insertion	Action(s)	Innervation
Digastric	Muscle with two bellies (anterior and posterior) linked by a tendon attached to the body and greater horn of the hyoid bone	Medial surface of the mastoid process of the temporal bone	Lower border of the mandible near the midline with the intermediate tendon tethered to the hyoid by a fibrous loop of connective tissue	With the mandible stabilized, aids in elevating the hyoid	**Posterior belly** Digastric branch of the facial nerve (cranial nerve VII) **Anterior belly** Mylohyoid branch of the inferior alveolar nerve of the mandibular division of the trigeminal (cranial nerve V)
Mylohyoid	Thin muscle forming the muscular "floor" of the oral cavity Deep to the digastric	Mylohyoid line on the internal surface of the mandible	**Posterior fibers** Body of the hyoid bone **Anterior fibers** Linked with fibers of the opposite side through the median raphe	Pulls hyoid superiorly	Mylohyoid branch of the inferior alveolar nerve of the mandibular division of the trigeminal (cranial nerve V)
Geniohyoid	Narrow, cylindrical muscle deep to the mylohyoid	Inferior mental spine on the internal surface of the mandible	Anterior surface of the body of the hyoid	Pulls hyoid anteriorly	First cervical spinal nerve (C1) traveling with fibers of the hypoglossal nerve (cranial nerve XII)
Stylohyoid	Long, thin muscle parallel to the posterior belly of the digastric	Styloid process of the temporal bone	Body of the hyoid bone near the greater horn	Elevates and retracts the hyoid bone	Stylohyoid branch of the facial nerve (cranial nerve VII)

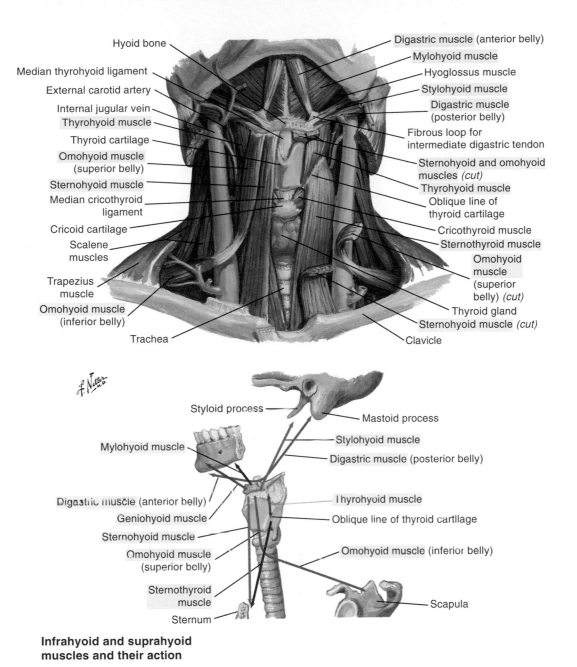

Hyoid bone

Median thyrohyoid ligament

External carotid artery

Internal jugular vein

Thyrohyoid muscle

Thyroid cartilage

Omohyoid muscle (superior belly)

Sternohyoid muscle

Median cricothyroid ligament

Cricoid cartilage

Scalene muscles

Trapezius muscle

Omohyoid muscle (inferior belly)

Trachea

Digastric muscle (anterior belly)

Mylohyoid muscle

Hyoglossus muscle

Stylohyoid muscle

Digastric muscle (posterior belly)

Fibrous loop for intermediate digastric tendon

Sternohyoid and omohyoid muscles (cut)

Thyrohyoid muscle

Oblique line of thyroid cartilage

Cricothyroid muscle

Sternothyroid muscle

Omohyoid muscle (superior belly) (cut)

Thyroid gland

Sternohyoid muscle (cut)

Clavicle

Styloid process

Mastoid process

Mylohyoid muscle

Stylohyoid muscle

Digastric muscle (posterior belly)

Digastric muscle (anterior belly)

Geniohyoid muscle

Sternohyoid muscle

Omohyoid muscle (superior belly)

Sternothyroid muscle

Sternum

Thyrohyoid muscle

Oblique line of thyroid cartilage

Omohyoid muscle (inferior belly)

Scapula

Infrahyoid and suprahyoid muscles and their action

Figure 2.10. The infrahyoid and suprahyoid muscles and their actions.

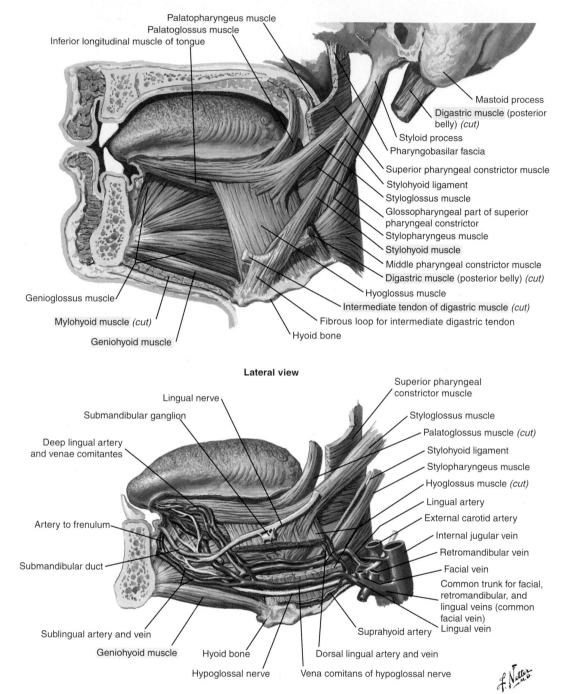

Palatopharyngeus muscle
Palatoglossus muscle
Inferior longitudinal muscle of tongue

Mastoid process
Digastric muscle (posterior belly) (cut)
Styloid process
Pharyngobasilar fascia
Superior pharyngeal constrictor muscle
Stylohyoid ligament
Styloglossus muscle
Glossopharyngeal part of superior pharyngeal constrictor
Stylopharyngeus muscle
Stylohyoid muscle
Middle pharyngeal constrictor muscle
Digastric muscle (posterior belly) (cut)
Hyoglossus muscle
Intermediate tendon of digastric muscle (cut)
Fibrous loop for intermediate digastric tendon

Genioglossus muscle
Mylohyoid muscle (cut)
Geniohyoid muscle
Hyoid bone

Lateral view

Lingual nerve
Submandibular ganglion
Deep lingual artery and venae comitantes
Artery to frenulum
Submandibular duct
Sublingual artery and vein
Geniohyoid muscle
Hypoglossal nerve

Superior pharyngeal constrictor muscle
Styloglossus muscle
Palatoglossus muscle (cut)
Stylohyoid ligament
Stylopharyngeus muscle
Hyoglossus muscle (cut)
Lingual artery
External carotid artery
Internal jugular vein
Retromandibular vein
Facial vein
Common trunk for facial, retromandibular, and lingual veins (common facial vein)
Lingual vein
Suprahyoid artery
Dorsal lingual artery and vein
Vena comitans of hypoglossal nerve
Hyoid bone

Figure 2.11. A lateral view of the tongue and surrounding muscles. Note the extrinsic muscles of the larynx.

OROPHARYNGEAL-ARTICULATORY SYSTEM

■ OVERVIEW

The supralaryngeal vocal tract is crucial for speech sound generation. Its function is to modify the laryngeal sound source to produce the sounds of speech. Vowels are created by changing the configuration of the vocal tract, which acts as a filter with modifiable resonant modes. Frequencies at or near these resonant modes (called *formant frequencies*) pass most effectively, whereas others are attenuated. Consequently, the frequency spectrum of the sound generated by the vibrating vocal folds is modified as it passes through the filter. The filter characteristics of the upper vocal tract depend on its shape, which is modified by movements of the articulators (e.g., tongue, jaw, and lips) through muscular action.

Consonants require rapid movements of one or more of the speech articulators to create transient or turbulent sound sources and may include an additional sound source from the vibrating vocal folds for voiced consonants. The nasal cavity is coupled (for nasalized sounds) or decoupled from the rest of the supralaryngeal vocal tract through the action of the velopharyngeal mechanism.

The same oropharyngeal-articulatory structures that participate in speech production are also vital for the manipulation and movement of food and liquids during mastication and swallowing.

This section focuses on the study of the oropharyngeal-articulatory system. First, cranial anatomy relative to the articulators and other associated structures of the vocal tract is discussed, followed by an examination of the various muscles of articulation and swallowing and their respective functions.

■ CRANIAL ANATOMY

The skull is an extremely complex osseous structure that provides protection for the brain (and middle and inner ears) and is the point of attachment of many muscles important for speech, mastication, and swallowing. The skull is composed of 22 bones (excluding the 6 middle ear ossicles), 8 paired and 6 unpaired. They are joined by sutures, which provide for growth in the developing skull, except for the mandible or lower jaw, which is the only movable cranial bone. In fact, the skull is sometimes divided into the cranium (which includes the facial skeleton) and the mandible. The cranium can be further divided into the *cranial vault,* the upper bowl-like portion that includes the skullcap or calvaria, and the *cranial base.* We will use the following main divisions of the skull:

1. The cranium (cranial skeleton), which is located in the superoposterior quadrant of the skull
2. The facial skeleton (including the mandible), which is located in the anteroinferior quadrant of the skull

Cranium (Figures 3.1, 3.2 [p. 112] and 3.3 [p. 113])

The cranium contains eight bones, four of which are unpaired.

Unpaired Bones

- The frontal bone contributes to the forehead, the anterior internal surface of the skull, the anterior cranial fossa, the orbit, and the nasal cavity.
- The occipital bone forms the posteroinferior margin of the cranial vault and contributes to the posterior cranial fossa. It encloses the foramen magnum, which is the point of communication between the brain and spinal cord.
- The sphenoid bone forms the pterygoid fossa located between the medial and lateral pterygoid plates. It contributes to the anterior and middle cranial fossae, the orbit, the temporal fossa, the infratemporal fossa, the pterygopalatine fossa, the scaphoid fossa, the nasal cavity, and the lateral wall of the cranial vault.
- The ethmoid bone contributes to the anterior cranial fossa, the lateral and superior walls of the nasal cavity, the nasal septum, and the medial wall of the orbital cavity.

Paired Bones

- Temporal bones contribute to the inferolateral margins of the cranial vault. They form the posterolateral part of the middle cranial fossa, the anterolateral part of the posterior cranial fossa, and the mandibular fossa; they also contain the middle and inner ear.
- Parietal bones contribute to the superior, lateral, and posterior portions of the cranial vault.

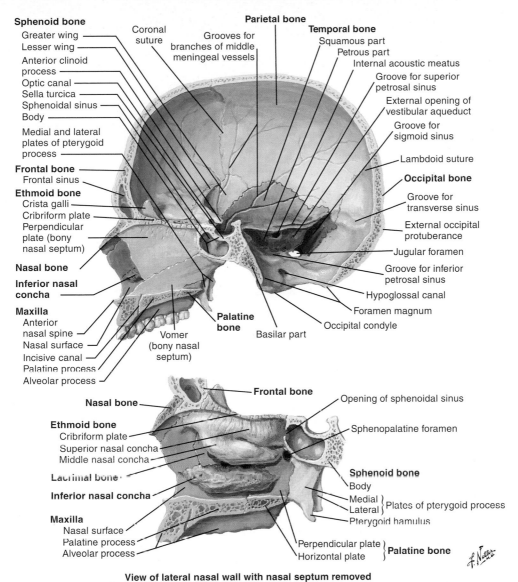

Sphenoid bone
Greater wing
Lesser wing
Anterior clinoid process
Optic canal
Sella turcica
Sphenoidal sinus
Body
Medial and lateral plates of pterygoid process

Frontal bone
Frontal sinus

Ethmoid bone
Crista galli
Cribriform plate
Perpendicular plate (bony nasal septum)

Nasal bone

Inferior nasal concha

Maxilla
Anterior nasal spine
Nasal surface
Incisive canal
Palatine process
Alveolar process

Coronal suture

Grooves for branches of middle meningeal vessels

Parietal bone

Temporal bone
Squamous part
Petrous part
Internal acoustic meatus
Groove for superior petrosal sinus
External opening of vestibular aqueduct
Groove for sigmoid sinus

Lambdoid suture

Occipital bone
Groove for transverse sinus
External occipital protuberance
Jugular foramen
Groove for inferior petrosal sinus
Hypoglossal canal
Foramen magnum
Occipital condyle

Palatine bone

Vomer (bony nasal septum)

Basilar part

Frontal bone

Nasal bone

Ethmoid bone
Cribriform plate
Superior nasal concha
Middle nasal concha

Lacrimal bone

Inferior nasal concha

Maxilla
Nasal surface
Palatine process
Alveolar process

Opening of sphenoidal sinus

Sphenopalatine foramen

Sphenoid bone
Body
Medial
Lateral } Plates of pterygoid process
Pterygoid hamulus

Perpendicular plate }
Horizontal plate } **Palatine bone**

View of lateral nasal wall with nasal septum removed

Figure 3.1. A midsagittal section of the cranium.

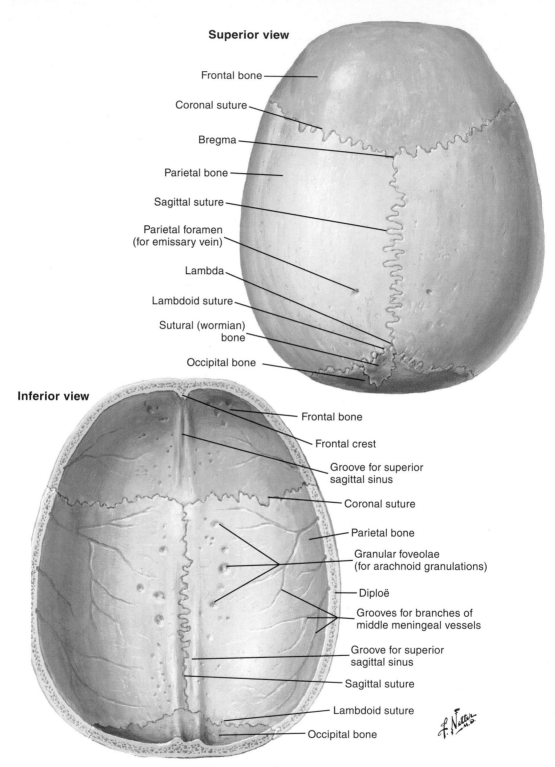

Superior view

Frontal bone

Coronal suture

Bregma

Parietal bone

Sagittal suture

Parietal foramen
(for emissary vein)

Lambda

Lambdoid suture

Sutural (wormian)
bone

Occipital bone

Inferior view

Frontal bone

Frontal crest

Groove for superior
sagittal sinus

Coronal suture

Parietal bone

Granular foveolae
(for arachnoid granulations)

Diploë

Grooves for branches of
middle meningeal vessels

Groove for superior
sagittal sinus

Sagittal suture

Lambdoid suture

Occipital bone

Figure 3.2. Superior and inferior views of the skullcap.

Frontal bone
  Groove for superior sagittal sinus
  Frontal crest
  Groove for anterior meningeal vessels
  Foramen cecum
  Superior surface of orbital part

Ethmoid bone
  Crista galli
  Cribriform plate

Sphenoid bone
  Lesser wing
    Anterior clinoid process
  Greater wing
    Groove for middle meningeal
    vessels (frontal branches)
  Body
    Jugum
    Prechiasmatic groove
  Sella turcica { Tuberculum sellae
                 Hypophyseal fossa
                 Dorsum sellae
                 Posterior clinoid process
  Carotid groove (for int. carotid a.)
  Clivus

Temporal bone
  Squamous part
  Petrous part
  Groove for lesser petrosal nerve
  Groove for greater petrosal nerve
  Arcuate eminence
  Trigeminal impression
  Groove for superior petrosal sinus
  Groove for sigmoid sinus

Parietal bone
  Groove for middle meningeal
  vessels (parietal branches)
  Mastoid angle

Occipital bone
  Clivus
  Groove for inferior petrosal sinus
  Basilar part
  Groove for posterior meningeal vessels
  Condyle
  Groove for transverse sinus
  Groove for occipital sinus
  Internal occipital crest
  Internal occipital protuberance
  Groove for superior sagittal sinus

Anterior cranial fossa

Middle cranial fossa

Posterior cranial fossa

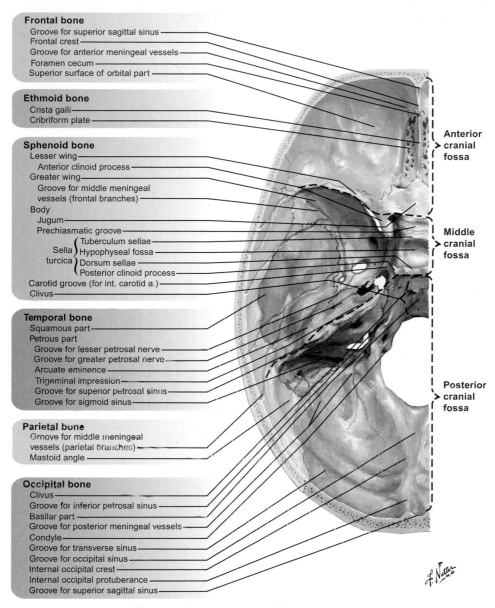

Figure 3.3. Superior view of the cranial base.

Facial Skeleton (Figures 3.4, 3.5 [p. 116], and 3.6 [p. 117])

The facial skeleton is constructed of 14 bones, 2 of which are unpaired.

Unpaired Bones of the Facial Skeleton

Mandible

The mandible forms the inferior border of the face and is composed of three parts: the horizontal body containing the alveolar process and the mandibular teeth and the two rami. On each ramus are the coronoid and condylar processes. The condylar processes articulate with the cranial temporal bones to form the temporomandibular joint (see p. 144).

Vomer

The vomer forms part of the bony nasal septum (with the perpendicular plate of the ethmoid) and the posterior wall of the nasal cavity.

Paired Bones of the Facial Skeleton

Maxilla

The maxilla is made up of two bones that join at the median line. They contribute to the upper jaw, cheek, infratemporal region, pterygopalatine fossa, floor of the orbit, palatal vault, and lateral wall and floor of the nasal cavity. Each bone has four processes: zygomatic, frontal, palatine, and alveolar (supporting the maxillary teeth).

Nasal Bones

Nasal bones contribute to the superior and lateral walls of the nasal cavity and the external "bridge" of the nose.

Palatine Bones

The palatine bones contribute to the lateral wall and floor of the nasal cavity, the oral cavity (more precisely, the posterior one-third of the hard palate), the pterygopalatine fossa, and the posterior wall of the orbit.

Lacrimal Bones

The lacrimal bones contribute to the medial wall of the orbit and the lateral wall of the nasal cavity.

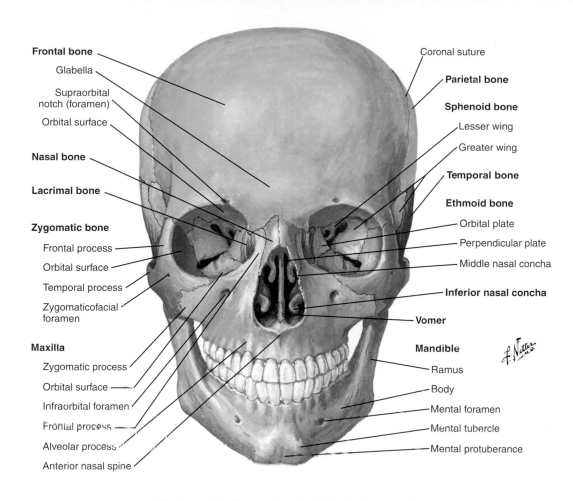

Frontal bone
Glabella
Supraorbital notch (foramen)
Orbital surface

Nasal bone

Lacrimal bone

Zygomatic bone
Frontal process
Orbital surface
Temporal process
Zygomaticofacial foramen

Maxilla
Zygomatic process
Orbital surface
Infraorbital foramen
Frontal process
Alveolar process
Anterior nasal spine

Coronal suture
Parietal bone
Sphenoid bone
Lesser wing
Greater wing
Temporal bone
Ethmoid bone
Orbital plate
Perpendicular plate
Middle nasal concha
Inferior nasal concha
Vomer
Mandible
Ramus
Body
Mental foramen
Mental tubercle
Mental protuberance

Right orbit: frontal and slightly lateral view

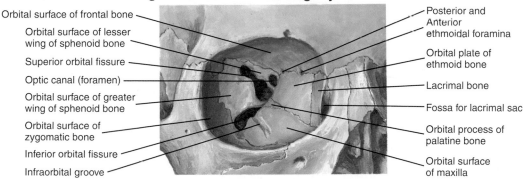

Orbital surface of frontal bone
Orbital surface of lesser wing of sphenoid bone
Superior orbital fissure
Optic canal (foramen)
Orbital surface of greater wing of sphenoid bone
Orbital surface of zygomatic bone
Inferior orbital fissure
Infraorbital groove

Posterior and Anterior ethmoidal foramina
Orbital plate of ethmoid bone
Lacrimal bone
Fossa for lacrimal sac
Orbital process of palatine bone
Orbital surface of maxilla

Figure 3.4. Anterior view of the skull and the facial skeleton.

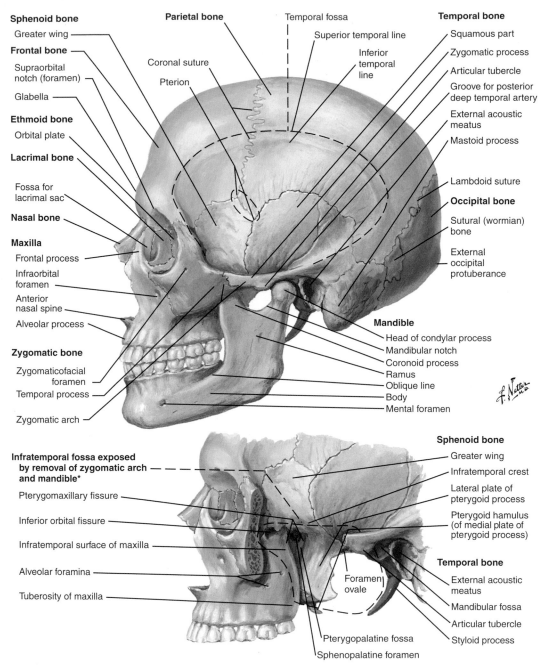

Sphenoid bone

Greater wing

Frontal bone

Supraorbital notch (foramen)

Glabella

Ethmoid bone

Orbital plate

Lacrimal bone

Fossa for lacrimal sac

Nasal bone

Maxilla

Frontal process

Infraorbital foramen

Anterior nasal spine

Alveolar process

Zygomatic bone

Zygomaticofacial foramen

Temporal process

Zygomatic arch

Parietal bone

Coronal suture

Pterion

Temporal fossa

Superior temporal line

Inferior temporal line

Temporal bone

Squamous part

Zygomatic process

Articular tubercle

Groove for posterior deep temporal artery

External acoustic meatus

Mastoid process

Lambdoid suture

Occipital bone

Sutural (wormian) bone

External occipital protuberance

Mandible

Head of condylar process

Mandibular notch

Coronoid process

Ramus

Oblique line

Body

Mental foramen

Infratemporal fossa exposed by removal of zygomatic arch and mandible*

Pterygomaxillary fissure

Inferior orbital fissure

Infratemporal surface of maxilla

Alveolar foramina

Tuberosity of maxilla

Foramen ovale

Pterygopalatine fossa

Sphenopalatine foramen

Sphenoid bone

Greater wing

Infratemporal crest

Lateral plate of pterygoid process

Pterygoid hamulus (of medial plate of pterygoid process)

Temporal bone

External acoustic meatus

Mandibular fossa

Articular tubercle

Styloid process

*Superficially, mastoid process forms posterior boundary.

Figure 3.5. Lateral view of the skull and the facial skeleton.

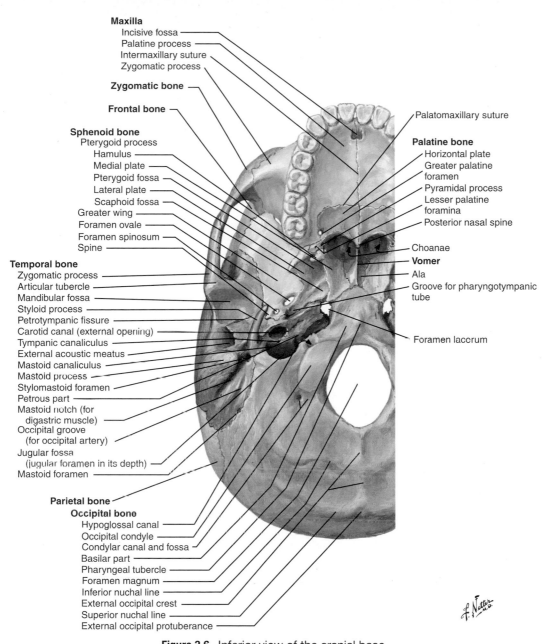

Maxilla
Incisive fossa
Palatine process
Intermaxillary suture
Zygomatic process

Zygomatic bone

Frontal bone

Sphenoid bone
Pterygoid process
Hamulus
Medial plate
Pterygoid fossa
Lateral plate
Scaphoid fossa
Greater wing
Foramen ovale
Foramen spinosum
Spine

Temporal bone
Zygomatic process
Articular tubercle
Mandibular fossa
Styloid process
Petrotympanic fissure
Carotid canal (external opening)
Tympanic canaliculus
External acoustic meatus
Mastoid canaliculus
Mastoid process
Stylomastoid foramen
Petrous part
Mastoid notch (for
    digastric muscle)
Occipital groove
    (for occipital artery)
Jugular fossa
    (jugular foramen in its depth)
Mastoid foramen

Parietal bone
Occipital bone
Hypoglossal canal
Occipital condyle
Condylar canal and fossa
Basilar part
Pharyngeal tubercle
Foramen magnum
Inferior nuchal line
External occipital crest
Superior nuchal line
External occipital protuberance

Palatomaxillary suture

Palatine bone
Horizontal plate
Greater palatine
    foramen
Pyramidal process
Lesser palatine
    foramina
Posterior nasal spine

Choanae
Vomer
Ala
Groove for pharyngotympanic
    tube

Foramen lacerum

Figure 3.6. Inferior view of the cranial base.

Zygomatic Bones

The zygomatic bones form the skeletal support of the cheek (thus the common name "cheekbone"). They contribute to the zygomatic arch, the lateral wall of the orbit, and the anterior wall of the infratemporal region.

Inferior Nasal Conchae

The inferior nasal conchae contribute to the formation of the lateral wall of the nasal cavity and the medial wall of the maxillary sinus.

Sinuses

Cranial and facial bones contain sinuses, which are air-filled cavities located near the nasal cavity, and are as follows:

- Maxillary sinus
- Frontal sinus
- Sphenoidal sinus
- Ethmoidal sinus

■ VOCAL TRACT

The vocal tract is the portion of the upper airway above the vocal folds and includes the pharyngeal, nasal, and oral cavities.

Pharyngeal Cavity or Pharynx (see Figures 3.7 [p. 120] and 3.8 [p. 121])

The pharynx is an musculomembranous tube that extends from the cranial base to the opening of the cervical esophagus which is located at the level of the inferior border of the cricoid cartilage (anteriorly) and of the sixth or seventh cervical vertebrae (posteriorly). Its inferior border is continuous with the cervical esophagus. Fibers of three circular constrictors and three longitudinal elevator muscles can be found in its lateral and posterior walls (for a detailed description of the pharyngeal muscles and their action, see "Muscles of the Pharynx" [pp. 155–159]; see also the section describing the palatopharyngeus muscle [p. 154]). The pharynx forms a part of the vocal tract and is involved in velopharyngeal closure (see p. 157). It is also importantly involved in the transportation of food and liquid for swallowing.

The pharynx is often divided into three portions:

1. The nasopharynx is located posterior to the posterior nasal apertures (choanae). It is bounded superiorly by the mucosa covering the body of the sphenoid and the basilar part of the occipital bone and inferiorly by the velum (soft palate). The nasopharynx has a roof, a posterior wall, and two lateral walls. Its floor (the velum) can be raised and lowered through soft palate muscle activation. An important mass of lymphatic tissue, the pharyngeal tonsils (adenoids), is located in the mucosa of the roof and posterior wall of the nasopharynx. Important surface features can also be found in the lateral walls and include the pharyngeal opening of the pharyngotympanic tube, the salpingopharyngeal fold and the torus levatorius (covering the salpingopharyngeus and levator veli palatine muscles, respectively), and the pharyngeal recess.

2. The oropharynx is posterior to the palatoglossal arch (or anterior faucial pillars). Its superior border is an imaginary line going from the inferior limit of the soft palate to the posterior wall, and its inferior border is an imaginary line going from the superior border of the epiglottis to the posterior wall. The palatopharyngeal arch (posterior faucial pillars) and palatine tonsils lie in the lateral walls of the oropharynx and the root of the tongue forms part of its anterior wall. The root of the tongue is attached to the epiglottis via the median and lateral glossoepiglottic folds. These folds delineate two depressions named *valleculae* located between the root of the tongue and the anterior surface of the epiglottis (see Figure 3.11 [p. 127]). The valleculae are important landmarks during modified barium swallow studies, as bolus residue can accumulate in the valleculae during swallowing.

3. The laryngopharynx (or hypopharynx) is posterior to the larynx. Its superior border is an imaginary line going from the superior border of the epiglottis to the posterior wall, and its inferior border is the opening of the cervical esophagus. The laryngeal inlet and the posterior surface of the cricoid and arytenoid cartilages are located in the anterior wall of the laryngopharynx. On each side of the laryngeal inlet, there is a pyriform sinus (fossa) (see Figure 3.8 [p. 121]), which is a small recess located between the aryepiglottic fold (medially) and the thyroid cartilage and thyrohyoid membrane (laterally). The pyriform sinuses are also important landmarks during modified barium swallow studies.

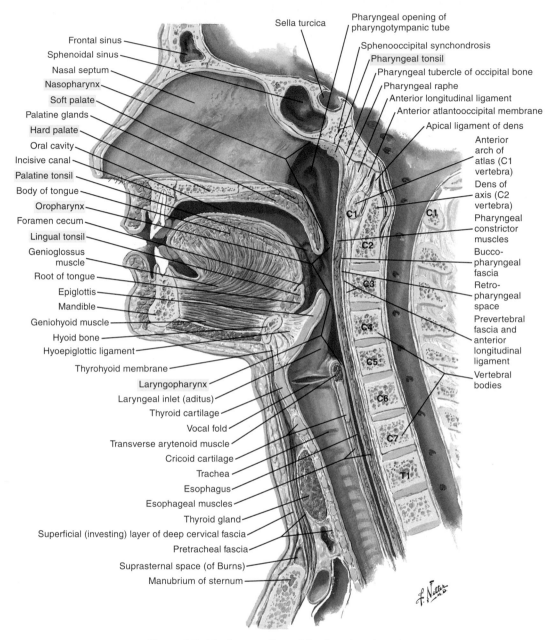

Figure 3.7. Median section of the head and neck.

Note Labels of certain figures are highlighted in yellow to emphasize the related elements in the corresponding text.

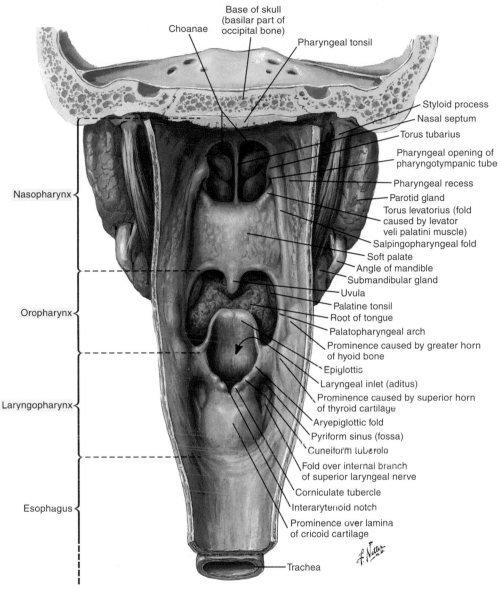

Choanae
Base of skull
(basilar part of
occipital bone)
Pharyngeal tonsil

Styloid process
Nasal septum
Torus tubarius
Pharyngeal opening of
pharyngotympanic tube
Pharyngeal recess
Parotid gland
Torus levatorius (fold
caused by levator
veli palatini muscle)
Salpingopharyngeal fold
Soft palate
Angle of mandible
Submandibular gland
Uvula
Palatine tonsil
Root of tongue
Palatopharyngeal arch
Prominence caused by greater horn
of hyoid bone
Epiglottis
Laryngeal inlet (aditus)
Prominence caused by superior horn
of thyroid cartilage
Aryepiglottic fold
Pyriform sinus (fossa)
Cuneiform tubercle
Fold over internal branch
of superior laryngeal nerve
Corniculate tubercle
Interarytenoid notch
Prominence over lamina
of cricoid cartilage

Nasopharynx
Oropharynx
Laryngopharynx
Esophagus

Trachea

Figure 3.8. Opened posterior view of the pharynx.

Nasal Cavity (Figure 3.9)

The nasal cavity is divided medially by the nasal septum, which has cartilaginous and osseous parts. The lateral walls are delineated by coiled, bony structures called *conchae* that are covered with mucous membranes. There are three conchae on each side: the superior, middle, and inferior nasal conchae. The conchae filter, moisten, and warm respired air. These convoluted structures increase surface area contact with the air.

During the production of non-nasal sounds of speech and for swallowing, the nasal cavity is isolated from the rest of the vocal tract by action of the velopharyngeal mechanism (see p. 157). The cartilages of the nasal cavity include the following:

- Septal cartilage
- Lateral cartilage
- Major alar cartilage
- Minor alar cartilage

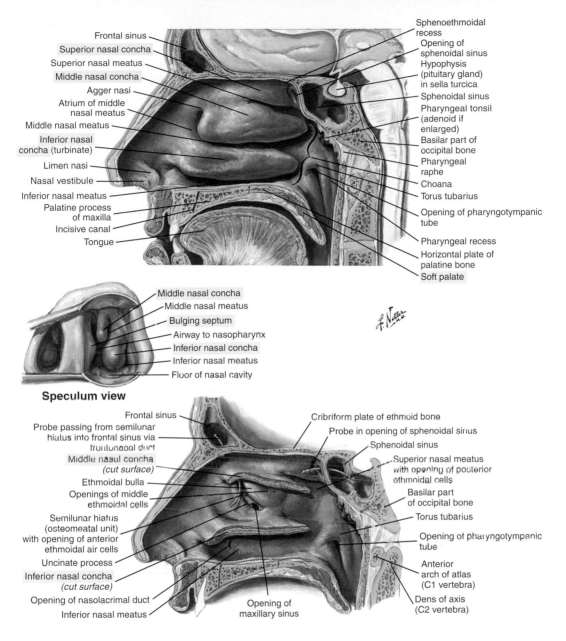

Figure 3.9. Lateral wall of the nasal cavity.

Frontal sinus
Superior nasal concha
Superior nasal meatus
Middle nasal concha
Agger nasi
Atrium of middle nasal meatus
Middle nasal meatus
Inferior nasal concha (turbinate)
Limen nasi
Nasal vestibule
Inferior nasal meatus
Palatine process of maxilla
Incisive canal
Tongue

Sphenoethmoidal recess
Opening of sphenoidal sinus
Hypophysis (pituitary gland) in sella turcica
Sphenoidal sinus
Pharyngeal tonsil (adenoid if enlarged)
Basilar part of occipital bone
Pharyngeal raphe
Choana
Torus tubarius
Opening of pharyngotympanic tube
Pharyngeal recess
Horizontal plate of palatine bone
Soft palate

Middle nasal concha
Middle nasal meatus
Bulging septum
Airway to nasopharynx
Inferior nasal concha
Inferior nasal meatus
Floor of nasal cavity

Speculum view

Frontal sinus
Probe passing from semilunar hiatus into frontal sinus via frontonasal duct
Middle nasal concha (cut surface)
Ethmoidal bulla
Openings of middle ethmoidal cells
Semilunar hiatus (osteomeatal unit) with opening of anterior ethmoidal air cells
Uncinate process
Inferior nasal concha (cut surface)
Opening of nasolacrimal duct
Inferior nasal meatus

Cribriform plate of ethmoid bone
Probe in opening of sphenoidal sinus
Sphenoidal sinus
Superior nasal meatus with opening of posterior ethmoidal cells
Basilar part of occipital bone
Torus tubarius
Opening of pharyngotympanic tube
Anterior arch of atlas (C1 vertebra)
Dens of axis (C2 vertebra)
Opening of maxillary sinus

Oral Cavity (Figure 3.10)

Delineation of the oral cavity is as follows:

- Anterior limit is the lips and teeth.
- Lateral limit is the cheeks and teeth.
- Posterior limit is the palatoglossal arch (or anterior faucial pillars).
- Superior limit is the palate.
- Inferior limit is the tongue and floor of the mouth.

Note that the delineation of the oral cavity varies considerably from one reference text to another.

The buccal space (oral vestibule), or cavity, represents the space between the lips and the teeth and between the cheeks and the teeth.

The articulators include the following (Figure 3.10):

- Lips
- Cheeks
- Teeth
- Mandible
- Tongue
- Hard palate
- Soft palate
- Pharynx

During an examination of the oral cavity, it is possible to see two pairs of folds located in the posterolateral part of the oral cavity, as follows:

1. The palatoglossal arch (or anterior faucial pillars) is formed by the palatoglossal muscle.
2. The palatopharyngeal arch (or posterior faucial pillars) is formed by the palatopharyngeus muscle.

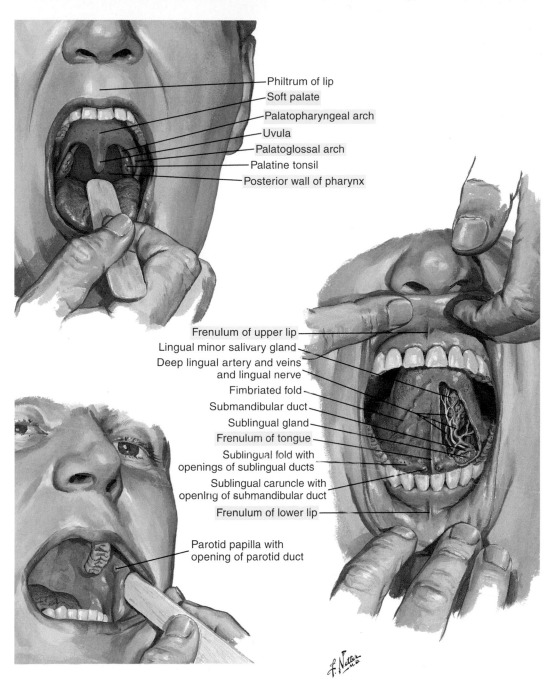

- Philtrum of lip
- Soft palate
- Palatopharyngeal arch
- Uvula
- Palatoglossal arch
- Palatine tonsil
- Posterior wall of pharynx

- Frenulum of upper lip
- Lingual minor salivary gland
- Deep lingual artery and veins and lingual nerve
- Fimbriated fold
- Submandibular duct
- Sublingual gland
- Frenulum of tongue
- Sublingual fold with openings of sublingual ducts
- Sublingual caruncle with opening of submandibular duct
- Frenulum of lower lip

- Parotid papilla with opening of parotid duct

Figure 3.10. Examination of the oral cavity.

Tonsils (Figure 3.11; see also Figure 3.7 [p. 120])

- Palatine tonsils, composed of lymphatic tissue, are located between the palatoglossal arch and the palatopharyngeal arch.
- Nasopharyngeal tonsils or pharyngeal tonsils (adenoids) are located on the roof and posterior wall of the nasopharynx.
- Tubal tonsils are located near the opening of the pharyngotympanic tube.
- Lingual tonsils cover the base of the tongue.

Together, these tonsils form the Waldeyer's tonsillar ring, which protects the body from infections.

Palate (see Figure 3.7 [p. 120])

The palate is the superior limit of the oral cavity and is composed of the following two parts:

- The hard palate is the osseous anterior two-thirds of the palate formed by the palatine processes of the maxilla (anteriorly) and the horizontal plates of the palatine bones (posteriorly).
- The soft palate or velum is a mobile structure forming the posterior one-third of the palate composed of connective tissue, muscular fibers, and mucosa.

At the posterior extremity of the palate, the uvula appears as an inferiorly directed projection of the posterior border of the soft palate.

Tongue (Figure 3.11)

The tongue is the primary articulator for speech sound production and is also crucial for oral bolus containment and the manipulation and transport of food and liquid during mastication and swallowing. The following landmarks can be observed on the tongue surface:

- Foramen cecum
- Terminal sulcus
- Median sulcus (midline groove)
- Circumvallate, foliate, filiform, and fungiform papillae
- Lingual tonsils

When looking at the underside of the tongue, it is possible to see a bridge of tissue on the median line that links the tongue to the mouth floor. This fold is called the *lingual frenulum* (frenulum of the tongue) (see Figures 3.10 [p. 125] and 3.12 [p. 129]).

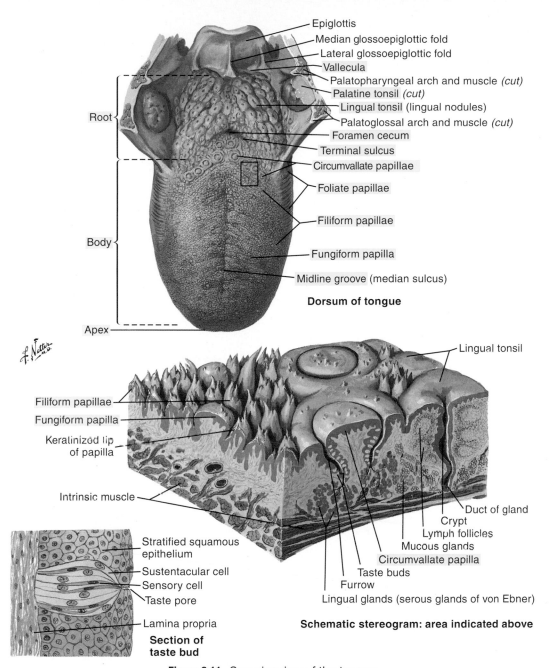

Dorsum of tongue

Epiglottis
Median glossoepiglottic fold
Lateral glossoepiglottic fold
Vallecula
Palatopharyngeal arch and muscle *(cut)*
Palatine tonsil *(cut)*
Lingual tonsil (lingual nodules)
Palatoglossal arch and muscle *(cut)*
Foramen cecum
Terminal sulcus
Circumvallate papillae
Foliate papillae
Filiform papillae
Fungiform papilla
Midline groove (median sulcus)

Root
Body
Apex

Lingual tonsil

Filiform papillae
Fungiform papilla
Keratinized lip
of papilla
Intrinsic muscle

Duct of gland
Crypt
Lymph follicles
Mucous glands
Circumvallate papilla
Taste buds
Furrow
Lingual glands (serous glands of von Ebner)

Stratified squamous
epithelium
Sustentacular cell
Sensory cell
Taste pore
Lamina propria

**Section of
taste bud**

Schematic stereogram: area indicated above

Figure 3.11. Superior view of the tongue.

Salivary Glands (Figure 3.12)

Saliva is extremely important for the breakdown and transport of food during mastication, taste, swallowing, and digestion. It is also crucial for oral health and as a lubricant for speech production and other oral motor activities. Saliva is produced by extrinsic and intrinsic salivary glands. There are three pairs of extrinsic salivary glands that produce the majority of the saliva. They are located outside but secrete into the oral cavity and are as follows:

1. Parotid glands
2. Submandibular glands
3. Sublingual glands

Lips (see Figure 3.10 [p. 125])

The lips are located at the anterior extremity of the oral cavity and are important for speech sound production and for oral bolus containment during mastication and swallowing. The external surface of the lips is covered by skin and the internal surface by mucous membrane. The tissue between these two layers (external and internal) is muscular, adipose, and glandular.

Looking at the external surface of the lips, the following are visible:

- The nasolabial fold (and associated crease, furrow, or sulcus) is a prominent fold from the lateral margin of the nose to the angle of the mouth.
- The labiomandibular fold extends from the corner of the mouth to the mandible. It is often seen as a continuation of the more superior nasolabial fold. Facial muscle contraction and movements of the nasolabial and labiomandibular folds (and associated creases) signal important facial expressions such as smiling.
- Philtral ridges are the two vertical parallel crests above the superior lip.
- The philtrum is the space between the philtral ridges.
- The mentolabial sulcus is between the lower lip and the chin.
- Cupid's bow is the well-defined border of the upper lip.
- Vermilion zones are the transition zones between the skin of the face and the mucous membrane that covers the internal surface of the upper and lower lips.
- The labial commissure is the angle or corner of the mouth.
- The modiolus is not visible on surface inspection but is located lateral to the labial commissure. There is one on each side of the mouth, and they are dense, mobile, approximately cone-shaped masses formed by the convergence of muscle fibers from several labial/facial muscles and other fibrous tissue. They are key anatomical structures for controlling movements of the lips for a variety of activities, including speech, mastication, swallowing, and facial expression.

The internal surface of the lips is covered by a mucous membrane with a thin and transparent epithelium. The pink color is the result of underlying vascularity.

Pulling up on the upper lip exposes the frenulum of the upper lip, which is the median tissue that links the lip to the maxilla. Pulling down on the lower lip exposes the frenulum of the lower lip, which is a median fold of tissue that links the lower lip to the mandible.

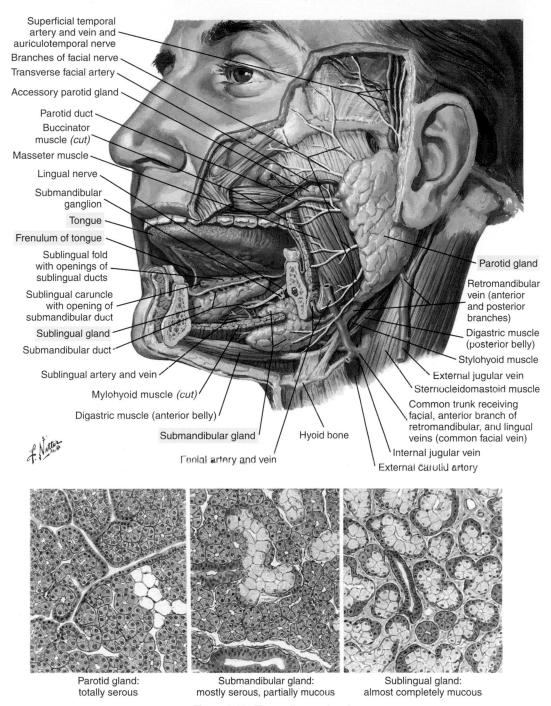

Superficial temporal artery and vein and auriculotemporal nerve
Branches of facial nerve
Transverse facial artery
Accessory parotid gland
Parotid duct
Buccinator muscle *(cut)*
Masseter muscle
Lingual nerve
Submandibular ganglion
Tongue
Frenulum of tongue
Sublingual fold with openings of sublingual ducts
Sublingual caruncle with opening of submandibular duct
Sublingual gland
Submandibular duct
Sublingual artery and vein
Mylohyoid muscle *(cut)*
Digastric muscle (anterior belly)
Submandibular gland
Facial artery and vein
Hyoid bone

Parotid gland
Retromandibular vein (anterior and posterior branches)
Digastric muscle (posterior belly)
Stylohyoid muscle
External jugular vein
Sternocleidomastoid muscle
Common trunk receiving facial, anterior branch of retromandibular, and lingual veins (common facial vein)
Internal jugular vein
External carotid artery

Parotid gland: totally serous

Submandibular gland: mostly serous, partially mucous

Sublingual gland: almost completely mucous

Figure 3.12. The salivary glands.

Teeth (Figures 3.13 and 3.14 [p. 132])

The teeth are speech articulators and importantly involved in mastication. They develop and emerge from alveolar processes of the mandible and maxilla. The alveoli are covered externally by the gingivae or gums, which are made of fibrous conjunctive tissue. A normal adult has 32 permanent teeth, which are as follows:

- 8 incisors
- 4 canines, or cuspids
- 8 premolars, or bicuspids
- 12 molars, including the third molars, commonly called *wisdom teeth*
  Each tooth is composed of the following:
- The crown is the portion of the tooth that extends above the alveolar boundary.
- The root is the portion of the tooth attached to the alveolar processes of the maxilla or mandible. The dental hole, or canal, located at the extremity of the root, allows for the dental nerves and the vessels.
- The cusp is the prominence on the occlusal surface of the tooth. Canines (also called *cuspids*) have one such prominence. Premolars (also called *bicuspids*) have two, and molars have four or five.

Surfaces are used to describe the external appearance of a tooth, and each tooth contains five surfaces, as follows:

1. The occlusal surface is the part of the tooth that is in contact with the tooth of the opposite jaw (maxilla or mandible).
2. The lingual surface is adjacent to the tongue.
3. The buccal surface is adjacent to the cheek for premolars and molars.
4. The labial surface is adjacent to the lips for incisors and canines.
5. The distal and mesial surfaces represent the sides of each tooth that are adjacent to other teeth in the same jaw (maxilla or mandible). The mesial surface is oriented anteriorly, and the distal surface is located posteriorly.

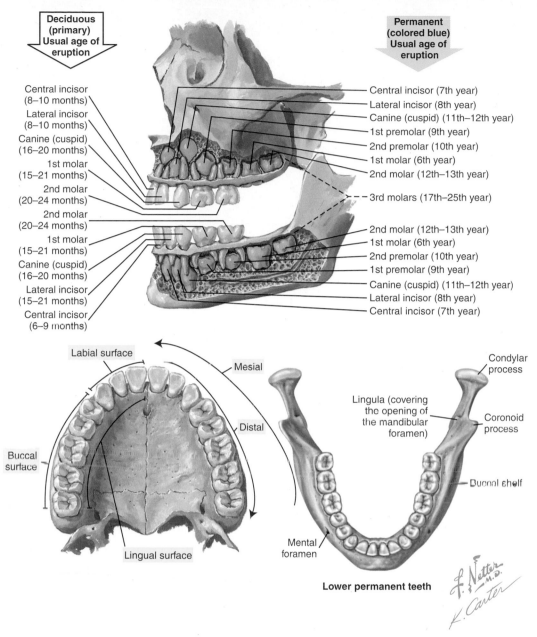

Deciduous (primary) Usual age of eruption

Central incisor (8–10 months)
Lateral incisor (8–10 months)
Canine (cuspid) (16–20 months)
1st molar (15–21 months)
2nd molar (20–24 months)
2nd molar (20–24 months)
1st molar (15–21 months)
Canine (cuspid) (16–20 months)
Lateral incisor (15–21 months)
Central incisor (6–9 months)

Permanent (colored blue) Usual age of eruption

Central incisor (7th year)
Lateral incisor (8th year)
Canine (cuspid) (11th–12th year)
1st premolar (9th year)
2nd premolar (10th year)
1st molar (6th year)
2nd molar (12th–13th year)
3rd molars (17th–25th year)
2nd molar (12th–13th year)
1st molar (6th year)
2nd premolar (10th year)
1st premolar (9th year)
Canine (cuspid) (11th–12th year)
Lateral incisor (8th year)
Central incisor (7th year)

Labial surface
Mesial
Buccal surface
Distal
Lingual surface

Condylar process
Lingula (covering the opening of the mandibular foramen)
Coronoid process
Buccal shelf
Mental foramen

Lower permanent teeth

Figure 3.13. Teeth: age of eruption and surfaces.

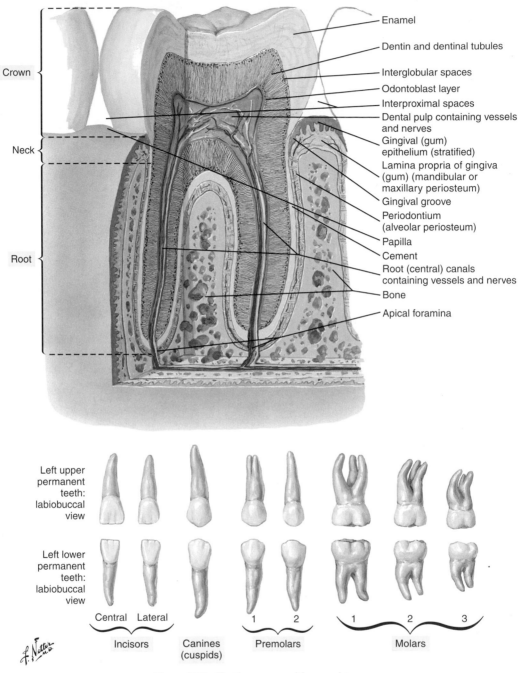

Figure 3.14. Teeth: composition and types.

Dental Occlusion

Globally, dental occlusion is the alignment and relationship between the teeth. Occlusion can also be defined as the normal contact between the occlusal surfaces of the teeth of the mandible and maxilla. The classification system of Dr. Edward H. Angle is often used, although not without controversy, to describe occlusal relationships between teeth. This system uses the relationship between the first molars of the mandible and maxilla and does not describe other potential problems with tooth alignment (e.g., crowding). Angle's system includes the following classifications:

- Class I neutral occlusion occurs when the first maxillary molar is slightly posterior and external to the first mandibular molar. More precisely, the mesiobuccal cusp of the first maxillary molar is aligned with the mesiobuccal groove (the one that separates the distal and mesial cusps) of the first mandibular molar.
- Class I malocclusion occurs when there is a neutral relationship between the molars, but there are problems with the alignment of anterior (mesial) teeth.
- Class II ("overbite") occurs when the first maxillary molar is anterior and external to the first mandibular molar or aligned with the first mandibular molar. More precisely, the mesiobuccal cusp of the first maxillary molar is anterior to the mesiobuccal groove (the one that separates the distal and mesial cusps) of the first mandibular molar. Class II is divided into the following:
  - Division I, in which the relationship between the central incisors is normal (i.e., the maxillary central incisors are in protrusion and slightly overhang the mandibular central incisors).
  - Division II, in which the relationship between the central incisors is abnormal (i.e., the maxillary central incisors, even if they are anterior to the mandibular incisors, are in retraction and inclined toward the tongue).
- Class III ("underbite") occurs when the first maxillary molar is significantly posterior to the first mandibular molar. More precisely, the mesiobuccal cusp of the first maxillary molar is posterior to the mesiobuccal groove (the one that separates the distal and mesial cusps) of the first mandibular molar.

■ MUSCLES OF THE LIPS AND FACIAL EXPRESSION

The muscles of the lips and facial expression are not always attached from bone to bone or bone to cartilage. Rather, many originate from a bone and insert on the skin or on other muscles. A complex orientation and interdigitation of lip muscle fibers underlie the synergistic actions of these muscles to generate the precise movements necessary for facial expression, social interaction, speech production, mastication, and swallowing. The considerable complexity of facial and lip musculature combined with variability in location and morphology across individuals (which may be the result of differences in facial size and shape) make exact determinations of muscle function difficult.

We will concentrate on muscles of the midface, lower face, and neck, and muscles will be classified in relationship to the orbicularis oris muscle, giving rise to transverse, angular, and vertical muscles.

Orbicularis Oris Muscle (Figures 3.15 and 3.16 [p. 137])

The orbicularis oris muscle is composed of primarily horizontally oriented muscle fibers that encircle the mouth in four quadrants: left, right, superior, and inferior, with each quadrant fanning out from the modiolus to the facial midline. Muscle fibers in each quadrant can be further delineated into a marginal portion (pars marginalis), deep to the vermilion, and a peripheral portion (pars peripheralis), around the lips.

Once thought to have a simple sphincter-like or constrictor function, our current understanding is of a much more complex muscle whose actions depend on the co-activation of other facial muscles. The orbicularis oris muscle is involved in lip compression for mastication, swallowing, and speech sound production.

The orbicularis oris muscle is innervated by the buccal and mandibular branches of the facial nerve (cranial nerve VII).

Two Transverse Muscles (Figures 3.15 and 3.16 [p. 137])

Buccinator Muscle

The buccinator muscle is a deep facial muscle and a primary muscle of the cheeks. To obtain a good view of this muscle, we have to remove the masseter, which is an important jaw-closing muscle. The buccinator is a quadrilateral muscle that originates from the pterygomandibular raphe (ligament) and the molar alveolar processes of the mandible and maxilla. Muscle fibers course anteriorly (horizontally) to insert into the modiolus and the superior and inferior portions of the orbicularis oris muscle (crossed and uncrossed fibers) at the angle of the mouth. Muscle contraction pulls the lips laterally (retraction), compresses the cheeks, and assists in manipulating the food bolus during mastication and swallowing.

The buccinator muscle is innervated by the buccal branch of the facial nerve (cranial nerve VII).

Risorius Muscle

The risorius muscle shows considerable individual variability and is often absent. It is parallel and superficial to the buccinator muscle. It originates from the fascia above the parotid gland and the aponeurosis of the masseter muscle and inserts into the modiolus. Muscular contraction pulls the lips laterally, as in laughing or smiling.

The risorius is innervated by the zygomatic and buccal branches of the facial nerve (cranial nerve VII).

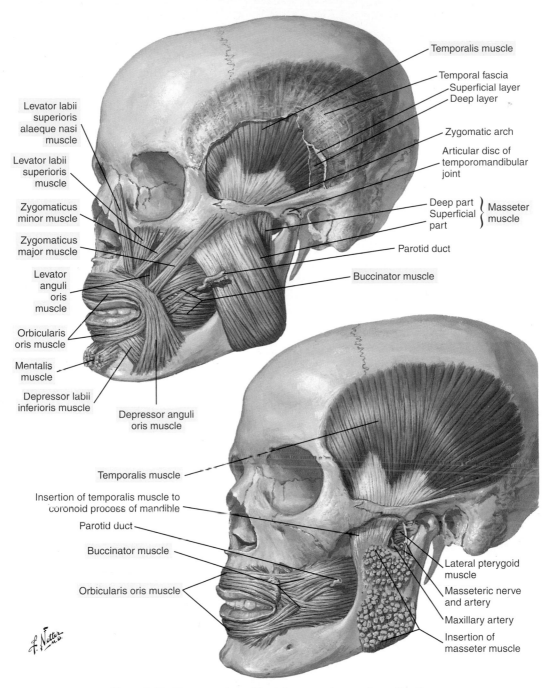

Figure 3.15. The muscles of facial expression and mastication.

Five Angular Muscles (Figure 3.16; see also Figure 3.15 [p. 135])

Levator Labii Superioris Alaeque Nasi Muscle

The levator labii superioris alaeque nasi muscle originates from the frontal process of the maxilla and divides into medial and lateral muscular portions. The medial portion inserts into the alar cartilage and acts to dilate the nostril. The lateral portion inserts into the lateral superior portion of the orbicularis oris muscle, elevates and everts (turns inside out) the upper lip, and contributes to deepening the nasolabial fold.

The levator labii superioris alaeque nasi muscle is innervated by the zygomatic and buccal branches of the facial nerve (cranial nerve VII).

Levator Labii Superioris Muscle

The levator labii superioris muscle originates lateral to the levator labii superioris alaeque nasi muscle from the inferior surface of the orbit to course inferiorly and medially to insert into the superior portion of the orbicularis oris muscle. It elevates and everts the upper lip and contributes to deepening the nasolabial fold.

The levator labii superioris muscle is innervated by the zygomatic and buccal branches of the facial nerve (cranial nerve VII).

Zygomaticus Minor Muscle

Sometimes absent, the zygomaticus minor muscle originates from the zygomatic bone lateral to the levator labii superioris and tracks inferiorly and medially to insert into the superior portion of the orbicularis oris muscle. Its action elevates the upper lip and contributes to deepening the nasolabial fold, as in smiling.

The zygomaticus minor muscle is innervated by the zygomatic and buccal branches of the facial nerve (cranial nerve VII).

Zygomaticus Major Muscle

The zygomaticus major muscle originates from the zygomatic bone, lateral to the zygomaticus minor muscle. It courses inferiorly and medially to insert into the superior portion of the orbicularis oris muscle and the modiolus. It is often composed of superficial and deep portions. Together with the levator anguli oris, its action pulls the lips superiorly and laterally such as when smiling or laughing.

The zygomaticus major muscle is innervated by the buccal and zygomatic branches of the facial nerve (cranial nerve VII).

Depressor Labii Inferioris Muscle

The depressor labii inferioris muscle originates from the external oblique line of the mandible. It travels superiorly and medially to insert into the modiolus and the inferior orbicularis oris muscle. Its action pulls the lower lip down during mastication and may also contribute to facial expressions such as sadness or sorrow.

The depressor labii inferioris muscle is innervated by the mandibular branch of the facial nerve (cranial nerve VII).

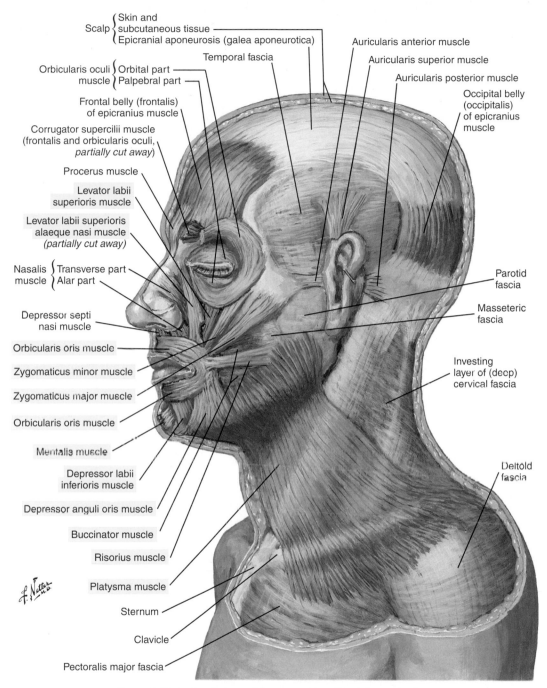

Scalp { Skin and subcutaneous tissue — Epicranial aponeurosis (galea aponeurotica)

Temporal fascia

Auricularis anterior muscle

Auricularis superior muscle

Auricularis posterior muscle

Occipital belly (occipitalis) of epicranius muscle

Orbicularis oculi muscle { Orbital part / Palpebral part —

Frontal belly (frontalis) of epicranius muscle

Corrugator supercilii muscle (frontalis and orbicularis oculi, *partially cut away*)

Procerus muscle

Levator labii superioris muscle

Levator labii superioris alaeque nasi muscle *(partially cut away)*

Nasalis muscle { Transverse part / Alar part

Depressor septi nasi muscle

Orbicularis oris muscle

Zygomaticus minor muscle

Zygomaticus major muscle

Orbicularis oris muscle

Mentalis muscle

Depressor labii inferioris muscle

Depressor anguli oris muscle

Buccinator muscle

Risorius muscle

Platysma muscle

Sternum

Clavicle

Pectoralis major fascia

Parotid fascia

Masseteric fascia

Investing layer of (deep) cervical fascia

Deltoid fascia

Figure 3.16. Lateral view of the muscles of facial expression.

Three Vertical Muscles (see Figures 3.15 [p. 135] and 3.16 [p. 137])

Mentalis Muscle

The mentalis muscle originates from the anterior surface of the body of the mandible to insert on the skin of the chin and on the inferior portion of the orbicularis oris muscle and the modiolus. Its action elevates, protrudes, and everts the lower lip and may crease the chin.

The mentalis muscle is innervated by the mandibular branch of the facial nerve (cranial nerve VII).

Levator Anguli Oris Muscle (Caninus)

The levator anguli oris muscle originates from the canine fossa of the maxilla to insert into the modiolus and the superior portion of the orbicularis oris muscle. As indicated by its name, its action elevates the angle of the mouth and, together with the zygomaticus major muscle, pulls the lips superiorly and laterally and deepens the nasolabial fold, as in smiling or laughing.

The levator anguli oris muscle is innervated by zygomatic and buccal branches of the facial nerve (cranial nerve VII).

Depressor Anguli Oris Muscle

The depressor anguli oris muscle partially covers and is lateral to the depressor labii inferioris muscle and is superficial to the platysma muscle. It originates from the external oblique line of the mandible and courses superiorly to insert into the modiolus and the inferior portion of the orbicularis oris muscle. Superiorly it is continuous with the levator anguli oris muscle and inferiorly with the platysma muscle. Its action depresses the angle of the mouth, as indicated by its name, such as in an expression of sadness.

The depressor anguli oris is innervated by the mandibular and buccal branches of the facial nerve (cranial nerve VII).

■ MUSCLE OF THE NECK

Platysma Muscle (see Figure 3.16 [p. 137])

The platysma muscle is very thin, flat, and large. It covers the majority of the anterior and lateral surfaces of the neck. Its extension is quite variable. It is deep to the depressor anguli oris muscle. In most individuals, it extends to the cheeks and the muscles of the mouth and the modiolus. However, for some, it can spread even farther up to the muscles surrounding the eyes. When this muscle contracts, it expands the neck and pulls the skin of the neck upward, which may also facilitate the drainage of nearby blood vessels. Also, this muscle may play a role in the downward movements of the lower lip and jaw.

The platysma is innervated by the cervical branch of the facial nerve (cranial nerve VII).

■ MUSCLES OF THE TONGUE

At a functional level, the tongue can be divided into the following sections (see Figure 3.11 [p. 127]):

The body constitutes the major mass of the tongue.

The root is the posterior portion that forms the anterior boundary of the pharyngeal cavity.

The dorsum is the dorsal surface of the tongue.

The blade is the anterior part of the tongue, just behind the apex and beneath the alveolar ridge of the maxilla.

The apex is the tip or the most anterior portion of the tongue.

These parts are particularly important for the tongue's actions for the production of the sounds of speech and for swallowing.

The tongue is composed of and controlled by the following two groups of muscles:

1. Intrinsic muscles have origins and insertions inside the tongue.
2. Extrinsic muscles have an origin outside the tongue and an insertion in the tongue.

Intrinsic Muscles of the Tongue (Figure 3.17)

The intrinsic muscles form a complex array of interdigitating muscle fibers. This complex arrangement allows for precise adjustments in tongue form and position. There are four intrinsic muscles, as follows:

1. Superior longitudinal muscle
2. Inferior longitudinal muscle
3. Transverse muscle
4. Vertical muscle

Horizontal section below lingula of mandible (superior view) demonstrating bed of parotid gland

Orbicularis oris muscle

Buccinator muscle

Buccopharyngeal fascia

Facial artery and vein

Pterygomandibular raphe

Lingual nerve and superior pharyngeal constrictor muscle

Masseter muscle

Palatoglossus muscle in palatoglossal arch

Palatine tonsil

Palatopharyngeus muscle in palatopharyngeal arch

Ramus of mandible

Inferior alveolar artery, vein, and nerve

Medial pterygoid muscle

Styloglossus muscle

Facial nerve

Retromandibular vein

External carotid artery

Parotid gland

Stylopharyngeus muscle

Stylohyoid muscle

Sternocleidomastoid muscle

Digastric muscle (posterior belly)

Internal jugular vein; internal carotid artery; and nerves IX, X, and XII in carotid sheath

Superior cervical sympathetic ganglion

Axis (C2)

Longus capitis muscle

Prevertebral fascia

Buccopharyngeal fascia and retropharyngeal space

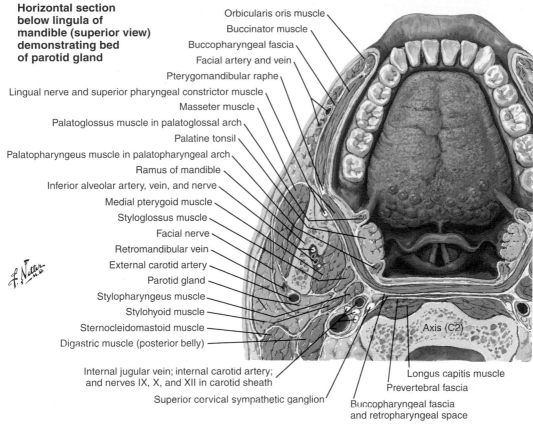

Superior longitudinal muscle

Vertical and transverse muscles } of tongue

Inferior longitudinal muscle

Styloglossus muscle

Buccinator muscle

Muscles of facial expression

Hyoglossus muscle

Genioglossus muscle

Sublingual salivary gland

Submandibular duct

Mandibular canal; inferior alveolar artery, vein, and nerve

Lingual nerve

Nerve to mylohyoid

Vena comitans of hypoglossal nerve (to lingual vein)

Lingual artery

Facial artery

Hypoglossal nerve (XII)

Submandibular salivary gland

Submandibular lymph node

Mylohyoid muscle

Facial vein

Intermediate digastric tendon

Platysma muscle

Hyoid bone

Frontal section behind 1st molar tooth (anterior view) demonstrating beds of sublingual and submandibular glands

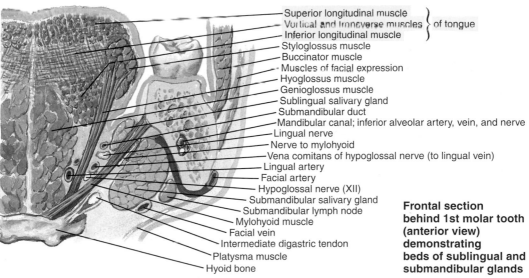

Figure 3.17. Superior view and coronal section of the tongue.

Extrinsic Muscles of the Tongue (Figure 3.18)

Extrinsic muscles link the tongue with surrounding structures. These muscles allow the tongue to move forward, backward, upward, downward, and laterally. Each name includes the word *glossus,* which means tongue, and another term indicating the external origin. There are four extrinsic muscles, as follows:

1. Palatoglossus muscle
2. Styloglossus muscle
3. Hyoglossus muscle
4. Genioglossus muscle

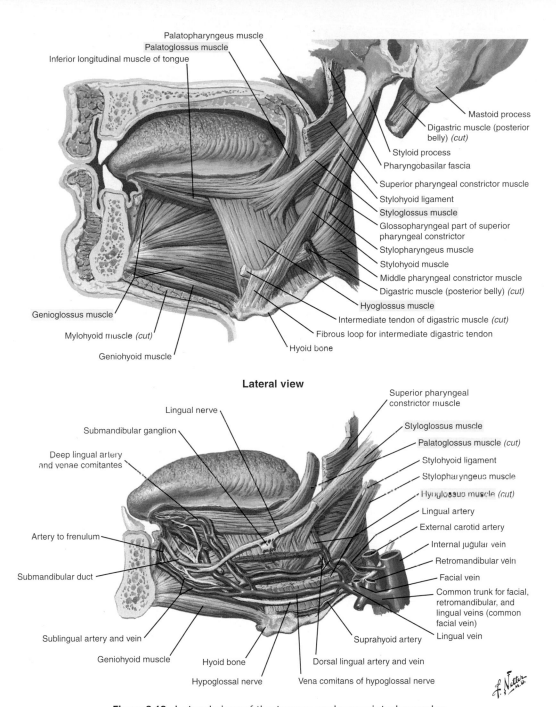

Palatopharyngeus muscle
Palatoglossus muscle
Inferior longitudinal muscle of tongue

Mastoid process
Digastric muscle (posterior belly) (cut)
Styloid process
Pharyngobasilar fascia
Superior pharyngeal constrictor muscle
Stylohyoid ligament
Styloglossus muscle
Glossopharyngeal part of superior pharyngeal constrictor
Stylopharyngeus muscle
Stylohyoid muscle
Middle pharyngeal constrictor muscle
Digastric muscle (posterior belly) (cut)
Hyoglossus muscle
Intermediate tendon of digastric muscle (cut)
Fibrous loop for intermediate digastric tendon

Genioglossus muscle
Mylohyoid muscle (cut)
Geniohyoid muscle
Hyoid bone

Lateral view

Lingual nerve
Submandibular ganglion
Deep lingual artery and venae comitantes

Superior pharyngeal constrictor muscle
Styloglossus muscle
Palatoglossus muscle (cut)
Stylohyoid ligament
Stylopharyngeus muscle
Hyoglossus muscle (cut)
Lingual artery
External carotid artery
Internal jugular vein
Retromandibular vein
Facial vein
Common trunk for facial, retromandibular, and lingual veins (common facial vein)
Lingual vein

Artery to frenulum
Submandibular duct

Sublingual artery and vein
Geniohyoid muscle
Hyoid bone
Hypoglossal nerve
Dorsal lingual artery and vein
Vena comitans of hypoglossal nerve
Suprahyoid artery

Figure 3.18. Lateral view of the tongue and associated muscles.

■ MUSCLES OF MASTICATION

Mastication is the process of food reduction and preparation for swallowing. It requires the complex coordinated movements of the jaw, lips, cheeks, and tongue. The origin of jaw muscles, often called *muscles of mastication,* is typically on the skull, and the insertion of jaw muscles is on the mandible, which is the movable portion of the jaw around the temporomandibular joint. Clearly, movements of the jaw are important for speech production, and as a result of biomechanical linkage, they influence the lips and the tongue. The muscles of mastication can generally be divided into jaw-opening and jaw-closing muscles, or jaw elevators and jaw depressors, respectively.

Temporomandibular Joint (Figure 3.19)

The temporomandibular joint is a synovial joint between the condylar process of the mandible and the anterior portion of the mandibular (articular, glenoid) fossa of the temporal bone. The articular surfaces of both structures are covered with fibrocartilage and separated by and connected to a cartilaginous articular disc. A fibrous articular capsule (joint capsule) surrounds these structures and thickens laterally to form the temporomandibular (lateral) ligament. This ligament courses from the mandible to the articular tubercle and zygomatic process of the temporal bone. Two other ligaments, the stylomandibular ligament and the sphenomandibular ligament, both located medially, may provide some additional support.

Two movements are associated with the temporomandibular joint, as follows:

1. Translation is a gliding type of movement that can be either bilateral (backward-forward movements of the jaw) or unilateral (the mandible moves from one side to the other).
2. Rotation is a "hinge-type" movement of the jaw. Imagine the jaw rotating around an imaginary horizontal axis through the condylar processes of the two sides of the mandible.

Mastication and speech involve a combination of these two types of jaw movements, with specific movement trajectories influenced by the nature of the food bolus and the timing within the masticatory sequence (from food ingestion to swallowing for mastication) and the specific speech sound produced and phonetic environment (for speech). There is also individual variability in both masticatory and speech movements.

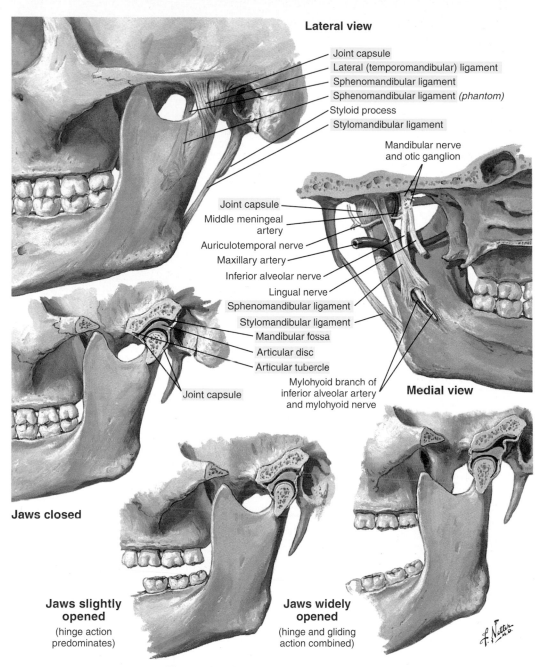

Lateral view

Joint capsule
Lateral (temporomandibular) ligament
Sphenomandibular ligament
Sphenomandibular ligament *(phantom)*
Styloid process
Stylomandibular ligament

Mandibular nerve
and otic ganglion

Joint capsule
Middle meningeal artery
Auriculotemporal nerve
Maxillary artery
Inferior alveolar nerve
Lingual nerve
Sphenomandibular ligament
Stylomandibular ligament
Mandibular fossa
Articular disc
Articular tubercle

Joint capsule

Mylohyoid branch of
inferior alveolar artery
and mylohyoid nerve

Medial view

Jaws closed

Jaws slightly opened
(hinge action predominates)

Jaws widely opened
(hinge and gliding action combined)

Figure 3.19. The temporomandibular joint.

Three Jaw-Closing Muscles (Jaw Elevators) (Figure 3.20; see also Figure 3.15 [p. 135])

Masseter Muscle

The masseter muscle has superficial (external) and deep (internal) fibers. The masseter muscle originates from the zygomatic process of the maxilla and the zygomatic arch. Fibers travel inferiorly to insert on the external surface of the angle and ramus of the mandible. Some fibers also insert on the coronoid process of the mandible. The masseter elevates the mandible. Superficial fibers may contribute to jaw protrusion and deep fibers to jaw retraction.

The masseter muscle is innervated by the masseter nerve of the mandibular division of the trigeminal nerve (cranial nerve V).

Temporalis Muscle

The temporalis muscle is composed of anterior, middle, and posterior portions. It originates from the temporal fossa on the frontal, parietal, temporal, and sphenoid bones. Its fibers converge under the zygomatic arch to form a tendon that inserts on the coronoid process and the anterior surface of the ramus of the mandible. Contraction of the anterior and middle portions of the temporalis muscle, composed principally of vertical fibers, elevates the mandible. Contraction of the posterior portion, which is made of more horizontal fibers, may elevate and retract the mandible. Unilateral contraction of these muscle fibers may contribute to lateral movements of the jaw.

The temporalis muscle is innervated by the deep temporal nerve of the mandibular division of the trigeminal nerve (cranial nerve V).

Medial (Internal) Pterygoid Muscle

The medial (internal) pterygoid muscle originates primarily from the medial surface of the lateral pterygoid plate of the sphenoid bone. A small group of fibers originates from the maxillary tuberosity and from the pyramidal process of the palatine bone. The fibers travel inferiorly, posteriorly, and laterally to insert on the internal surface of the angle and ramus of the mandible. This muscle forms, with the masseter muscle, a sling that surrounds the angle of the mandible and works with the masseter muscle and temporalis muscle to elevate the jaw. It acts in synergy with the lateral pterygoid muscle and the masseter muscle for jaw protrusion. Unilateral contraction of the medial pterygoid muscle moves the mandible laterally toward the opposite side. This action permits grinding movements during mastication.

The medial pterygoid muscle is innervated by the medial pterygoid nerve of the mandibular division of the trigeminal nerve (cranial nerve V).

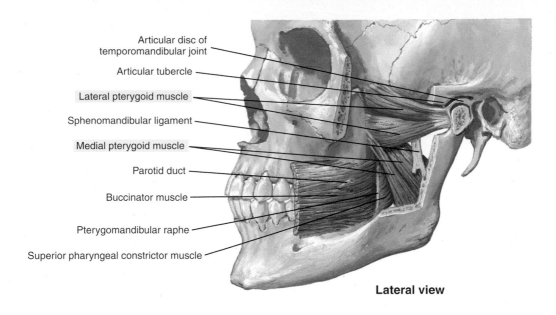

Articular disc of temporomandibular joint
Articular tubercle
Lateral pterygoid muscle
Sphenomandibular ligament
Medial pterygoid muscle
Parotid duct
Buccinator muscle
Pterygomandibular raphe
Superior pharyngeal constrictor muscle

Lateral view

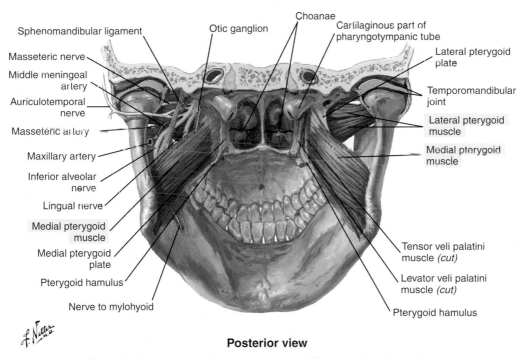

Sphenomandibular ligament
Masseteric nerve
Middle meningeal artery
Auriculotemporal nerve
Masseteric artery
Maxillary artery
Inferior alveolar nerve
Lingual nerve
Medial pterygoid muscle
Medial pterygoid plate
Pterygoid hamulus
Nerve to mylohyoid

Otic ganglion
Choanae
Cartilaginous part of pharyngotympanic tube
Lateral pterygoid plate
Temporomandibular joint
Lateral pterygoid muscle
Medial pterygoid muscle
Tensor veli palatini muscle (cut)
Levator veli palatini muscle (cut)
Pterygoid hamulus

Posterior view

Figure 3.20. Lateral and posterior views of the muscles of mastication.

Four Jaw-Opening Muscles (Jaw Depressors) (Figures 3.21 [p. 150] and 3.22 [p. 151]; see also Figure 3.20 [p. 147])

Lateral (External) Pterygoid Muscle

The lateral (external) pterygoid muscle has two heads. The superior portion originates from the fossa of the greater wing of the sphenoid bone and the inferior portion from the external surface of the lateral pterygoid plate of the sphenoid bone. Fibers course horizontally to insert on the articular disc of the temporomandibular joint and on the condylar process of the mandible. The superior portion of this muscle is co-activated with jaw-closing muscles during mastication. The bilateral contraction of the inferior portion protrudes the mandible. The alternating unilateral contraction of the inferior portion produces a lateral movement of the mandible toward the opposite side.

The lateral pterygoid muscle is innervated by the anterior trunk of the mandibular division of the trigeminal nerve (cranial nerve V).

Digastric Muscle

The digastric muscle is frequently classified as a suprahyoid muscle. Anatomically, this muscle contains posterior and anterior "bellies" (hence its name) that are linked by a central tendon. This central tendon is fixed to the hyoid bone by a loop-shaped intermediate tendon. With the jaw fixed by other muscles, muscular contraction may contribute to the elevation of the hyoid bone. With the hyoid bone fixed by the infrahyoid muscles, the digastric muscle acts as a jaw opener.

The posterior belly of the digastric muscle is innervated by the digastric branch of the facial nerve (cranial nerve VII), and the anterior belly of the digastric muscle is innervated by the mylohyoid branch of the inferior alveolar nerve of the mandibular division of the trigeminal nerve (cranial nerve V).

Mylohyoid Muscle

The mylohyoid muscle originates from the mylohyoid line (internal oblique line) of the mandible. The anterior and middle fibers insert into the median raphe joined by muscular fibers of the opposite side. The posterior fibers insert on the hyoid bone. The mylohyoid is fan-shaped and contributes to the muscular floor of the mouth. Contraction elevates the hyoid and the floor of the mouth (or stabilizes the floor). It can also contribute to jaw opening if the hyoid bone is fixed.

The mylohyoid muscle is innervated by the mylohyoid branch of the inferior alveolar nerve of the mandibular division of the trigeminal nerve (cranial nerve V).

Geniohyoid Muscle

The geniohyoid muscle extends from the internal surface of the mandible (inferior mental spine) to the hyoid bone. Two bellies are located on each side of the median line and almost parallel to the anterior bellies of the digastric muscle, which are inferior. Contraction of the mylohyoid and the geniohyoid muscles may retract the jaw. Their contraction also contributes to jaw opening if the hyoid bone is stabilized.

The geniohyoid muscle is innervated by the first cervical spinal nerve (C1) traveling with the fibers of the hypoglossal nerve (cranial nerve XII).

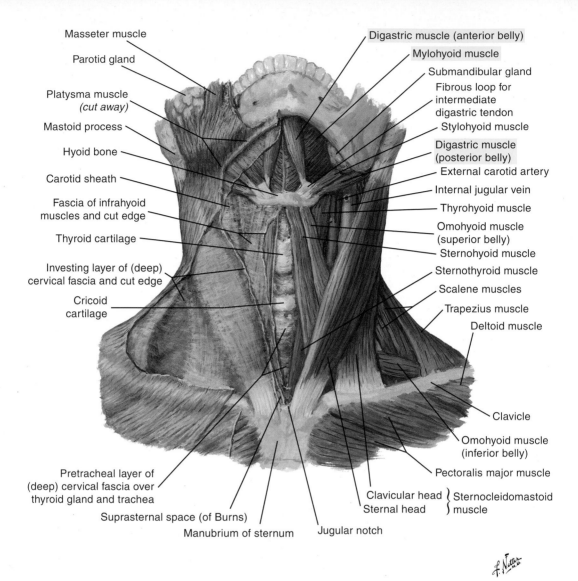

Masseter muscle

Parotid gland

Platysma muscle
(cut away)

Mastoid process

Hyoid bone

Carotid sheath

Fascia of infrahyoid
muscles and cut edge

Thyroid cartilage

Investing layer of (deep)
cervical fascia and cut edge

Cricoid
cartilage

Pretracheal layer of
(deep) cervical fascia over
thyroid gland and trachea

Suprasternal space (of Burns)

Manubrium of sternum

Jugular notch

Digastric muscle (anterior belly)

Mylohyoid muscle

Submandibular gland

Fibrous loop for
intermediate
digastric tendon

Stylohyoid muscle

Digastric muscle
(posterior belly)

External carotid artery

Internal jugular vein

Thyrohyoid muscle

Omohyoid muscle
(superior belly)

Sternohyoid muscle

Sternothyroid muscle

Scalene muscles

Trapezius muscle

Deltoid muscle

Clavicle

Omohyoid muscle
(inferior belly)

Pectoralis major muscle

Clavicular head } Sternocleidomastoid
Sternal head   } muscle

Figure 3.21. Anterior view of the neck. Note the digastric and the mylohyoid muscles, both jaw openers.

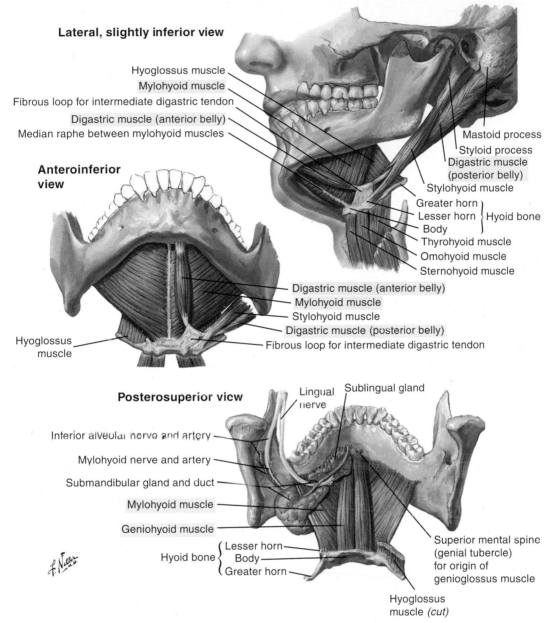

Lateral, slightly inferior view

Hyoglossus muscle
Mylohyoid muscle
Fibrous loop for intermediate digastric tendon
Digastric muscle (anterior belly)
Median raphe between mylohyoid muscles

Mastoid process
Styloid process
Digastric muscle (posterior belly)
Stylohyoid muscle
Greater horn ⎫
Lesser horn ⎬ Hyoid bone
Body ⎭
Thyrohyoid muscle
Omohyoid muscle
Sternohyoid muscle

Anteroinferior view

Hyoglossus muscle

Digastric muscle (anterior belly)
Mylohyoid muscle
Stylohyoid muscle
Digastric muscle (posterior belly)
Fibrous loop for intermediate digastric tendon

Posterosuperior view

Lingual nerve
Sublingual gland

Inferior alveolar nerve and artery
Mylohyoid nerve and artery
Submandibular gland and duct
Mylohyoid muscle
Geniohyoid muscle
Hyoid bone { Lesser horn
Body
Greater horn

Superior mental spine (genial tubercle) for origin of genioglossus muscle

Hyoglossus muscle (cut)

Figure 3.22. The floor of the mouth and three muscles contributing to jaw opening: (1) the digastric, (2) the mylohyoid, and (3) the geniohyoid.

■ MUSCLES OF THE SOFT PALATE

The soft palate, or velum, is a posterior extension of the hard or bony palate. It is formed principally by five muscles: the levator veli palatini, the tensor veli palatini, the palatoglossus, the palatopharyngeus, and the uvular. The only intrinsic muscle of the soft palate is the uvular muscle. All other muscles have an exterior attachment.

Levator Veli Palatini Muscle (Figure 3.23; see also Figure 3.8 [p. 121])

The levator veli palatini muscle is a palatal elevator. Fibers originate from the petrous portion of the temporal bone and the inferior aspect of the cartilaginous pharyngotympanic tube. Fibers travel inferiorly and toward the midline to insert into the palatine raphe (aponeurosis) of the soft palate. Contraction of this muscle pulls the soft palate toward the posterior pharyngeal wall. The role of this muscle in contributing to the opening of the pharyngotympanic tube for the ventilation of the middle ear is controversial.

The levator veli palatini muscle is innervated by the pharyngeal branch of the vagus nerve (cranial nerve X) via the pharyngeal plexus.

Tensor Veli Palatini Muscle (Figure 3.23)

The tensor veli palatini muscle has three origins: the scaphoid fossa of the medial pterygoid plate, the spine of the sphenoid bone, and the lateral cartilaginous walls of the pharyngotympanic tube. The fibers travel forward and downward to converge on a tendon that wraps around the hamulus and inserts into the palatine raphe (aponeurosis) and the horizontal plates of the palatine bone. This muscle dilates the pharyngotympanic tube and may also tense the palate.

The tensor veli palatini muscle is innervated by the medial pterygoid nerve of the mandibular division of the trigeminal nerve (cranial nerve V).

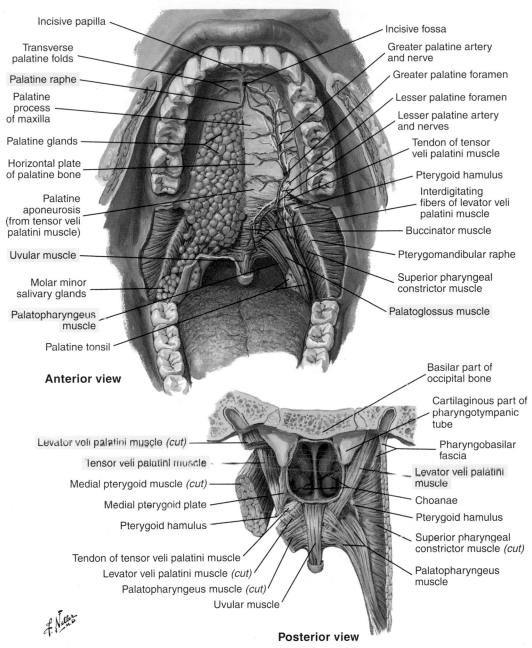

Incisive papilla

Transverse palatine folds

Palatine raphe

Palatine process of maxilla

Palatine glands

Horizontal plate of palatine bone

Palatine aponeurosis (from tensor veli palatini muscle)

Uvular muscle

Molar minor salivary glands

Palatopharyngeus muscle

Palatine tonsil

Anterior view

Incisive fossa

Greater palatine artery and nerve

Greater palatine foramen

Lesser palatine foramen

Lesser palatine artery and nerves

Tendon of tensor veli palatini muscle

Pterygoid hamulus

Interdigitating fibers of levator veli palatini muscle

Buccinator muscle

Pterygomandibular raphe

Superior pharyngeal constrictor muscle

Palatoglossus muscle

Levator veli palatini muscle (cut)

Tensor veli palatini muscle

Medial pterygoid muscle (cut)

Medial pterygoid plate

Pterygoid hamulus

Tendon of tensor veli palatini muscle

Levator veli palatini muscle (cut)

Palatopharyngeus muscle (cut)

Uvular muscle

Basilar part of occipital bone

Cartilaginous part of pharyngotympanic tube

Pharyngobasilar fascia

Levator veli palatini muscle

Choanae

Pterygoid hamulus

Superior pharyngeal constrictor muscle (cut)

Palatopharyngeus muscle

Posterior view

Figure 3.23. The soft palate and associated structures.

Palatoglossus (Glossopalatine) Muscle (see Figure 3.23 [p. 153])

The palatoglossus (glossopalatine) muscle originates from the inferior surface of the palatine raphe (aponeurosis). Fibers course inferiorly to insert underneath the sides of the posterior portion of the tongue, principally on superficial muscles (located under the posterior portions of the sides of the tongue) and transverse muscles. The muscular fibers of the palatoglossus muscle form the bulk of the palatoglossal arch (or anterior faucial pillars) visible in the oral cavity. Contraction of this muscle may depress the soft palate or elevate the tongue when the soft palate is fixed. This muscle approximates the palatoglossal arches.

The palatoglossus muscle is innervated by the pharyngeal branch of the vagus nerve (cranial nerve X) via the pharyngeal plexus.

Palatopharyngeus Muscle (see Figure 3.23 [p. 153])

The palatopharyngeus muscle originates from the palatine raphe (aponeurosis). Its fibers form the bulk of the palatopharyngeal arch (or posterior faucial pillars) visible in the oral cavity. Fibers travel inferiorly with the muscular fibers of the stylopharyngeus muscle. The palatopharyngeus muscle inserts on the posterior border of the thyroid cartilage and on the inferior portion of the pharynx. Contraction of this muscle may depress the soft palate, elevate and constrict the pharynx, and elevate the larynx. This muscle approximates the palatopharyngeal arches.

The palatopharyngeus muscle is innervated by the pharyngeal branch of the vagus nerve (cranial nerve X) via the pharyngeal plexus.

Uvular Muscle (Musculus Uvulae) (see Figure 3.23 [p. 153])

The uvular muscle extends from the posterior nasal spine and the palatine raphe (aponeurosis) to insert into the mucosa of the uvula. The function of this muscle is not well understood. However, it may play a role in the elevation of the soft palate. The uvula is an important landmark during an oral examination because its orientation and form may reflect anomalies of the hard and soft palate.

The uvular muscle is innervated by the pharyngeal branch of the vagus nerve (cranial nerve X) via the pharyngeal plexus.

■ MUSCLES OF THE PHARYNX

Superior Pharyngeal Constrictor Muscle (Figure 3.24 [p. 156])

The superior pharyngeal constrictor muscle forms a tube starting at the level of the pterygomandibular raphe. Its fibers circle around posteriorly to insert into the median pharyngeal raphe. This muscle forms the sides and the back of the nasopharynx and a part of the posterior wall of the oropharynx. Contraction of this muscle pulls the pharyngeal wall forward and reduces the pharyngeal diameter during swallowing, thus contributing to the contraction (or propulsive) pressure applied to the swallowed bolus. It also contributes to pharyngeal tone and plays a role in velopharyngeal closure, which is discussed on p. 157.

The superior constrictor muscle is innervated by the pharyngeal branch of the vagus nerve (cranial nerve X) via the pharyngeal plexus.

Middle Pharyngeal Constrictor Muscle (Figure 3.24 [p. 156])

The middle pharyngeal constrictor muscle originates from the greater horns of the hyoid bone and the stylohyoid ligament to circle posteriorly to insert in the median pharyngeal raphe. Its contraction reduces the diameter of the pharynx and contributes to the contraction (or propulsive) pressure applied to the swallowed bolus. It also contributes to pharyngeal tone.

The middle constrictor muscle is innervated by the pharyngeal branch of the vagus nerve (cranial nerve X) via the pharyngeal plexus.

Inferior Pharyngeal Constrictor Muscle (Figure 3.24 [p. 156])

The inferior pharyngeal constrictor muscle exerts the most force of the pharyngeal constrictors.

Some fibers originate from the thyroid lamina and insert on the median pharyngeal raphe to form the thyropharyngeus. Contraction of this muscle reduces the diameter of the inferior part of the pharynx.

Another part originates from the sides of the cricoid cartilage to form the cricopharyngeus muscle. This muscle is approximately 1 cm in length and is one of the primary components of the pharyngoesophageal segment (see p. 160). A myotomized and residual form of this muscle and the pharynx are used to generate the esophageal sound source used by patients with laryngectomies. Swallowed air is expelled against a closed pharyngoesophageal segment, causing it to vibrate.

The inferior constrictor muscle is innervated by the pharyngeal branch of the vagus nerve (cranial nerve X) via the pharyngeal plexus and by the recurrent laryngeal nerve and external branch of the superior laryngeal nerve of the vagus nerve.

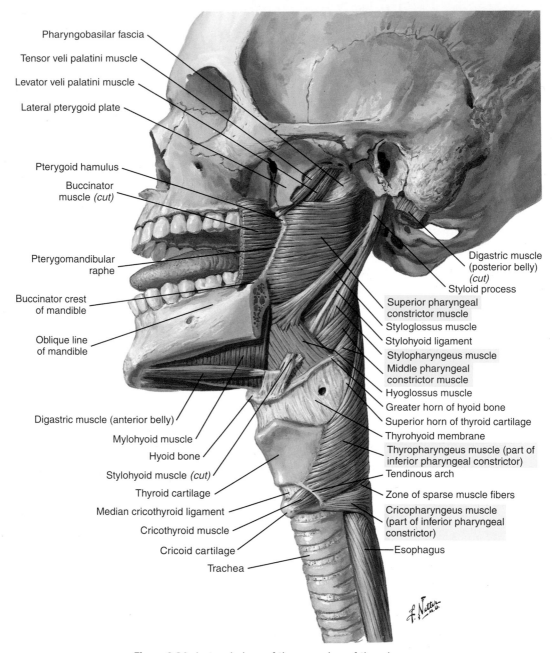

Pharyngobasilar fascia

Tensor veli palatini muscle

Levator veli palatini muscle

Lateral pterygoid plate

Pterygoid hamulus

Buccinator
muscle *(cut)*

Pterygomandibular
raphe

Buccinator crest
of mandible

Oblique line
of mandible

Digastric muscle (anterior belly)

Mylohyoid muscle

Hyoid bone

Stylohyoid muscle *(cut)*

Thyroid cartilage

Median cricothyroid ligament

Cricothyroid muscle

Cricoid cartilage

Trachea

Digastric muscle
(posterior belly)
(cut)

Styloid process

Superior pharyngeal
constrictor muscle

Styloglossus muscle

Stylohyoid ligament

Stylopharyngeus muscle

Middle pharyngeal
constrictor muscle

Hyoglossus muscle

Greater horn of hyoid bone

Superior horn of thyroid cartilage

Thyrohyoid membrane

Thyropharyngeus muscle (part of
inferior pharyngeal constrictor)

Tendinous arch

Zone of sparse muscle fibers

Cricopharyngeus muscle
(part of inferior pharyngeal
constrictor)

Esophagus

Figure 3.24. Lateral view of the muscles of the pharynx.

Salpingopharyngeus Muscle (Figure 3.25 [p. 158])

The salpingopharyngeus muscle originates at the inferoposterior surface of the cartilage of the pharyngotympanic tube and travels inferiorly and posteriorly to insert on the lateral walls of the pharynx. Its fibers mix with those of the palatopharyngeus muscle. Its contraction contributes to the elevation of the pharynx during swallowing and may contribute to the distortion of the tubal cartilage of the pharyngotympanic tube to permit aeration of the middle ear.

The salpingopharyngeus muscle is innervated by the pharyngeal branch of the vagus nerve (cranial nerve X) via the pharyngeal plexus.

Stylopharyngeus Muscle (Figure 3.26 [p. 159]; see also Figure 3.24 [p. 156])

The stylopharyngeus muscle constitutes a thin group of muscular fibers. Its origin is on the base of the styloid process of the temporal bone. It travels inferiorly and medially between the superior and middle pharyngeal constrictor muscles. This muscle inserts in the mucous membrane of the pharynx and on the thyroid cartilage. Its contraction elevates the larynx and elevates and expands the pharynx during swallowing.

The stylopharyngeus muscle is innervated by the glossopharyngeal nerve (cranial nerve IX).

Velopharyngeal Mechanism

The velopharyngeal mechanism is an essential process for speech and swallowing. It involves the movement of many oropharyngeal-articulatory structures that act to modify the coupling between the nasal and oral cavities. Some speech sounds are produced with the laryngeal voice source passing only through the oral cavity, excluding the nasal cavity (oral sounds), and some are produced with both the oral and nasal cavities (nasal sounds). The velopharyngeal mechanism acts as a regulator for coupling or decoupling of the nasal cavity from the rest of the vocal tract. Elevating and retracting the soft palate and moving the lateral walls of the nasopharynx medially and the posterior wall of the pharynx anteriorly (velopharyngeal closure) blocks the nasal cavity for the production of oral sounds. Opposite movements allow the laryngeal sound source to pass through and thus be modified by the nasal cavity. This creates the nasal sounds.

The velopharyngeal mechanism is also important for airway protection during mastication and swallowing. Closure prevents food from entering the nasal cavity during the passage of the bolus through the pharynx. Depression of the soft palate assists in containing the food and/or liquid bolus within the oral cavity before transport to the pharynx.

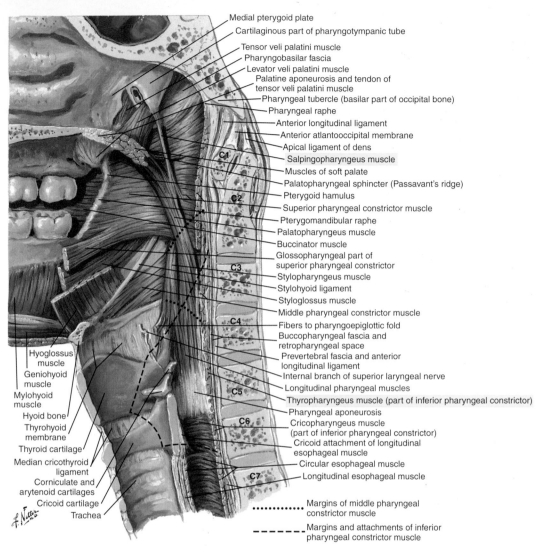

Medial pterygoid plate
Cartilaginous part of pharyngotympanic tube
Tensor veli palatini muscle
Pharyngobasilar fascia
Levator veli palatini muscle
Palatine aponeurosis and tendon of
tensor veli palatini muscle
Pharyngeal tubercle (basilar part of occipital bone)
Pharyngeal raphe
Anterior longitudinal ligament
Anterior atlantooccipital membrane
Apical ligament of dens
Salpingopharyngeus muscle
Muscles of soft palate
Palatopharyngeal sphincter (Passavant's ridge)
Pterygoid hamulus
Superior pharyngeal constrictor muscle
Pterygomandibular raphe
Palatopharyngeus muscle
Buccinator muscle
Glossopharyngeal part of
superior pharyngeal constrictor
Stylopharyngeus muscle
Stylohyoid ligament
Styloglossus muscle
Middle pharyngeal constrictor muscle
Fibers to pharyngoepiglottic fold
Buccopharyngeal fascia and
retropharyngeal space
Prevertebral fascia and anterior
longitudinal ligament
Internal branch of superior laryngeal nerve
Longitudinal pharyngeal muscles
Thyropharyngeus muscle (part of inferior pharyngeal constrictor)
Pharyngeal aponeurosis
Cricopharyngeus muscle
(part of inferior pharyngeal constrictor)
Cricoid attachment of longitudinal
esophageal muscle
Circular esophageal muscle
Longitudinal esophageal muscle

Hyoglossus
muscle
Geniohyoid
muscle
Mylohyoid
muscle
Hyoid bone
Thyrohyoid
membrane
Thyroid cartilage
Median cricothyroid
ligament
Corniculate and
arytenoid cartilages
Cricoid cartilage
Trachea

C1
C2
C3
C4
C5
C6
C7

•••••••••••• Margins of middle pharyngeal
constrictor muscle
– – – – – – Margins and attachments of inferior
pharyngeal constrictor muscle

Figure 3.25. Median (sagittal) section of the pharynx. Note especially the salpingopharyngeus muscle.

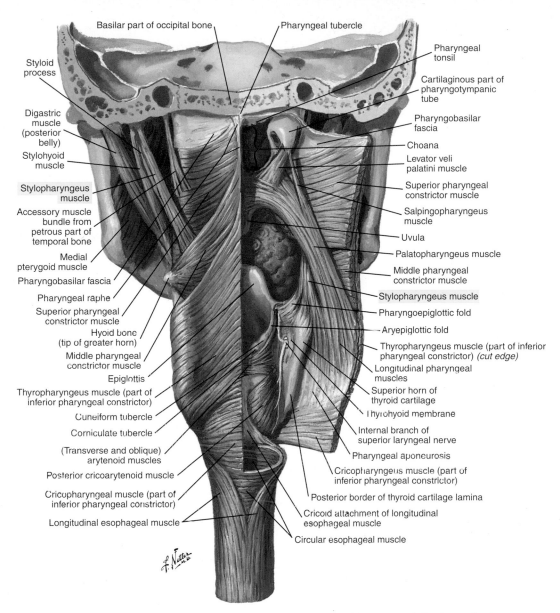

Figure 3.26. A posterior, partially reflected view of the pharynx. Note especially the stylopharyngeus muscle.

■ ESOPHAGUS

The esophagus is an important muscular tube that is approximately 25 cm in length. It is involved in transporting solids and liquids from the pharynx to the stomach during swallowing. It can be divided into three primary sections: cervical, thoracic, and abdominal esophagus. This complex structure is briefly summarized here.

Pharyngoesophageal Segment or Upper Esophageal Sphincter (Figures 3.27, 3.28 [p. 162], and 3.29 [p. 163])

The pharyngoesophageal segment is located at the junction of the laryngopharynx and esophagus. It is approximately 2.5 to 4.5 cm in length and extends from the level of the fourth cervical vertebra to the seventh. The term *upper esophageal sphincter* is often used to designate this segment, as it acts as a sphincter-like opening to the cervical esophagus. The muscular elements of this segment are the cricopharyngeus muscle and adjacent portions of the thyropharyngeus (part of the inferior pharyngeal constrictor muscle) and cervical esophageal musculature. The pharyngoesophageal segment is closed at rest primarily because of the tonic contraction of the cricopharyngeus, which prevents gastroesophageal reflux from entering the airway and prevents air from entering the esophagus. Relaxation of the cricopharyngeus muscle and laryngeal elevation by suprahyoid muscles "pulls away" the cricoid from the posterior pharyngeal wall and opens the pharyngoesophageal segment to allow liquids and solids to enter the esophagus from the pharynx during swallowing.

Primary Esophageal Peristalsis (see Figures 3.28 [p. 162] and 3.29 [p. 163])

Peristalsis is the process by which liquids or solids move through the esophagus by muscular contraction. It occurs subsequent to pharyngeal contraction and the opening of the pharyngoesophageal segment. Contractions in striated (cervical) esophageal muscle (inner circular and outer longitudinal fibers) are followed by smooth (thoracic) muscular contractions. Secondary peristalsis may clear bolus residue.

Lower Esophageal Sphincter (Figure 3.27)

The lower esophageal sphincter is the muscular junction between the esophagus and the stomach. It is closed to prevent gastroesophageal reflux by smooth esophageal muscle and crural portions of the diaphragm. The sphincter opens to accommodate the passage of the swallowed bolus into and out of the esophagus.

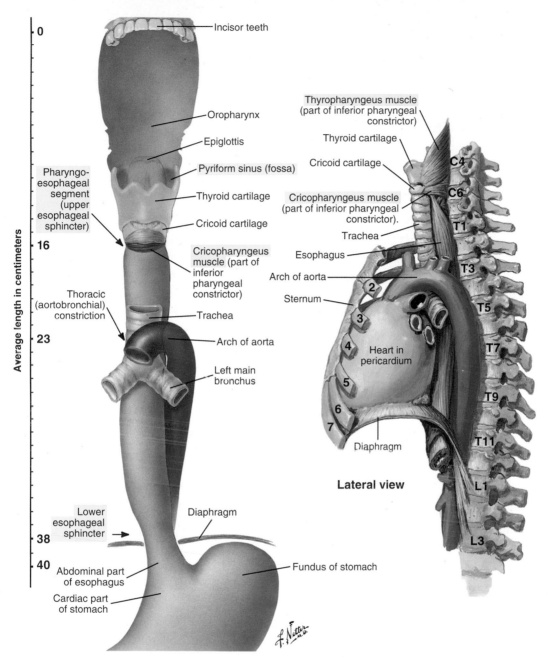

Figure 3.27. Topography and constrictions of the esophagus.

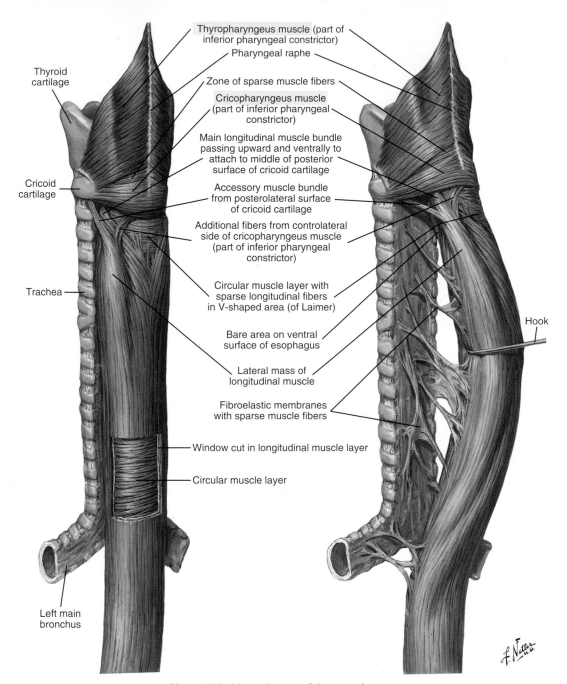

Thyropharyngeus muscle (part of inferior pharyngeal constrictor)

Pharyngeal raphe

Thyroid cartilage

Zone of sparse muscle fibers

Cricopharyngeus muscle (part of inferior pharyngeal constrictor)

Main longitudinal muscle bundle passing upward and ventrally to attach to middle of posterior surface of cricoid cartilage

Cricoid cartilage

Accessory muscle bundle from posterolateral surface of cricoid cartilage

Additional fibers from controlateral side of cricopharyngeus muscle (part of inferior pharyngeal constrictor)

Circular muscle layer with sparse longitudinal fibers in V-shaped area (of Laimer)

Trachea

Bare area on ventral surface of esophagus

Lateral mass of longitudinal muscle

Hook

Fibroelastic membranes with sparse muscle fibers

Window cut in longitudinal muscle layer

Circular muscle layer

Left main bronchus

Figure 3.28. Musculature of the esophagus.

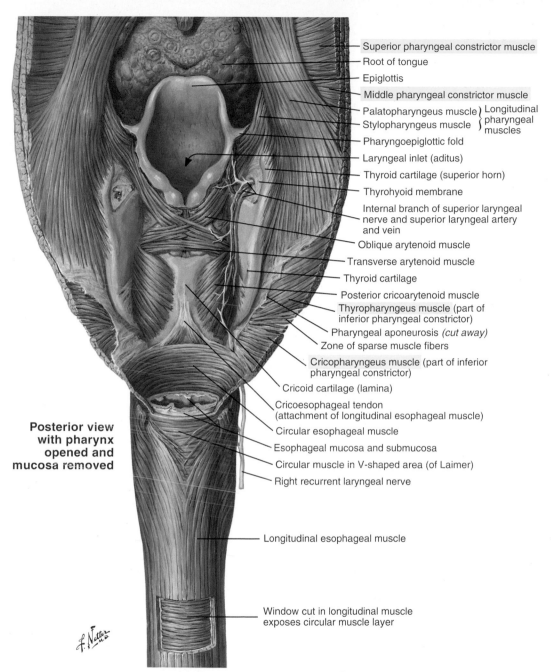

Superior pharyngeal constrictor muscle
Root of tongue
Epiglottis
Middle pharyngeal constrictor muscle
Palatopharyngeus muscle } Longitudinal
Stylopharyngeus muscle } pharyngeal muscles
Pharyngoepiglottic fold
Laryngeal inlet (aditus)
Thyroid cartilage (superior horn)
Thyrohyoid membrane
Internal branch of superior laryngeal nerve and superior laryngeal artery and vein
Oblique arytenoid muscle
Transverse arytenoid muscle
Thyroid cartilage
Posterior cricoarytenoid muscle
Thyropharyngeus muscle (part of inferior pharyngeal constrictor)
Pharyngeal aponeurosis *(cut away)*
Zone of sparse muscle fibers
Cricopharyngeus muscle (part of inferior pharyngeal constrictor)
Cricoid cartilage (lamina)
Cricoesophageal tendon (attachment of longitudinal esophageal muscle)
Circular esophageal muscle
Esophageal mucosa and submucosa
Circular muscle in V-shaped area (of Laimer)
Right recurrent laryngeal nerve
Longitudinal esophageal muscle
Window cut in longitudinal muscle exposes circular muscle layer

Posterior view with pharynx opened and mucosa removed

Figure 3.29. The pharyngoesophageal junction.

■ VISUALIZATION OF OROPHARYNGEAL-ARTICULATORY STRUCTURES

Several procedures make it possible to visualize vocal tract structures. These include naso-endoscopy, which uses a flexible tube inserted through the nose, attached to a camera, to obtain views of the pharynx and larynx. Nasoendoscopy is an important tool for assessing the vocal folds, the velopharyngeal mechanism, and swallowing.

Videofluoroscopy (also known as *modified barium swallow study*) is another procedure that captures high-resolution x-ray images of head and neck structures. This procedure is used to assess swallowing. Barium added to food or liquids is used as a contrast medium in this examination so that it can be seen as it moves through the pharynx and esophagus. Figure 3.30 is a static high-resolution x-ray image obtained from a videofluoroscopic swallowing examination (without bolus), illustrating the anatomical structures that can be observed in that view.

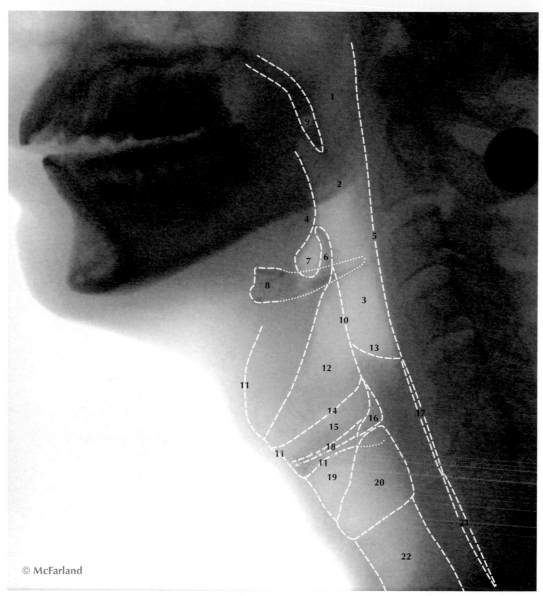

1. Nasopharynx	**9.** Soft palate	**17.** Pharyngoesophageal segment
2. Oropharynx	**10.** Aryepiglottic folds	**18.** Vocal folds
3. Laryngopharynx	**11.** Thyroid cartilage	**19.** Conus elasticus
4. Root of tongue	**12.** Laryngeal vestibule	**20.** Cricoid cartilage
5. Posterior wall of the pharynx	**13.** Pyriform sinuses	**21.** Esophagus
6. Epiglottis	**14.** Vestibular folds	**22.** Trachea
7. Valleculae	**15.** Laryngeal ventricule	
8. Hyoid bone	**16.** Arytenoid cartilages	

Figure 3.30. High-resolution x-ray image of the head and neck obtained from a videofluoroscopic swallowing study of a 60-year-old man. Important anatomical landmarks have been outlined in dotted lines and numbered. The solid black circle is a coin (a U.S. cent) used as a reference marker for distance measurements in scientific research.

Muscles of the Lips and Facial Expression (see Figures 3.15 [p. 135] and 3.16 [p. 137])

Muscles	Origin	Insertion	Action(s)	Innervation
Muscles of the Lips				
Orbicularis oris	Primarily horizontally oriented muscular fibers encircling the mouth from the modiolus	Facial midline	Complex function depends on other co-activated muscles: • Closes the lips and projects them forward • Contracts and presses the lips against the incisors	Buccal and mandibular branches of the facial nerve (cranial nerve VII)
Depressor anguli oris	External oblique line of the mandible	Modiolus and inferior portion of the orbicularis oris muscle	Depresses the angle of the mouth, as in a sad expression	Mandibular and buccal branches of the facial nerve (cranial nerve VII)
Levator anguli oris	Canine fossa of the maxilla	Modiolus and superior portion of the orbicularis oris muscle	Pulls the corner of the lips superiorly and laterally and deepens the nasolabial fold, as in smiling or laughing	Zygomatic and buccal branches of the facial nerve (cranial nerve VII)
Zygomaticus major	Zygomatic bone	Superior portion of the orbicularis oris muscle and modiolus	Pulls the lips superiorly and laterally, as when smiling or laughing	Buccal and zygomatic branches of the facial nerve (cranial nerve VII)
Risorius (variable muscle that is sometimes absent)	Fascia above the parotid gland Aponeurosis of the masseter muscle	Modiolus	Pulls the lips laterally, as in laughing	Zygomatic and buccal branches of the facial nerve (cranial nerve VII)
Levator labii superioris alaeque nasi	Frontal process of the maxilla	Medial portion: alar cartilage Lateral portion: superior portion of the orbicularis oris muscle	Medial portion: dilates nostril Lateral portion: elevates and everts the upper lip and contributes to deepen the nasolabial fold	Zygomatic and buccal branches of the facial nerve (cranial nerve VII)
Levator labii superioris	Inferior surface of orbit	Superior portion of the orbicularis oris muscle	Elevates and everts the upper lip and contributes to deepen the nasolabial fold	Zygomatic and buccal branches of the facial nerve (cranial nerve VII)
Depressor labii inferioris	External oblique line of the mandible	Modiolus and inferior portion of the orbicularis oris muscle	Pulls the lower lip down and may contribute to expressions of sadness	Mandibular branch of the facial nerve (cranial nerve VII)

Muscle	Origin	Insertion	Action	Innervation
Zygomaticus minor (variable muscle that is sometimes absent)	Zygomatic bone	Superior portion of orbicularis oris muscle and modiolus	Elevates the upper lip and deepens the nasolabial fold, as in smiling	Zygomatic and buccal branches of the facial nerve (cranial nerve VII)
Muscle of the Cheek				
Buccinator	Alveolar processes of the mandible and maxilla and pterygomandibular raphe; fibers course horizontally	Modiolus and superior and inferior portion of the orbicularis oris muscle	Compresses the cheeks / Pulls the lips laterally	Buccal branch of the facial nerve (cranial nerve VII)
Muscle of the Chin				
Mentalis	Anterior surface of the body of the mandible	Skin of the chin / Inferior portion of the orbicularis oris muscle / Modiolus	Elevates, protrudes, and everts the lower lip / May crease the chin	Mandibular branch of the facial nerve (cranial nerve VII)
Muscles of the Nose				
Nasalis compressor naris	Maxilla	Bridge of the nose	Compresses the back of the nose	Zygomatic and buccal branches of the facial nerve (cranial nerve VII)
Nasalis dilator naris	Nasal side of the maxillary bone	Alae of the nose	Dilates the nostrils	Zygomatic and buccal branches of the facial nerve (cranial nerve VII)
Depressor septi	Maxillary incisive fossa	Alae of the nose	Dilates the nostrils	Zygomatic and buccal branches of the facial nerve (cranial nerve VII)
Muscle of the Neck				
Platysma	Fascia covering the deltoid muscle and the pectoralis muscle	Cheeks and muscles of the mouth and modiolus / Some fibers may extend to muscles surrounding eyes (extent is variable)	Expands neck, pulls skin of neck upward, and depresses the lower lip and jaw	Cervical branch of the facial nerve (cranial nerve VII)

Muscles of the Tongue (see Figures 3.17 [p. 141] and 3.18 [p. 143])

Muscles	Origin	Insertion	Action(s)	Innervation
Intrinsic Tongue Muscles				
Superior longitudinal	Fibrous tissue at the root and median fibrous septum	Fibrous membrane on the sides of the tongue	Shortens the tongue Turns the apex upward	Hypoglossal nerve (cranial nerve XII)
Inferior longitudinal	Root of the tongue	Apex of the tongue	Shortens the tongue Pulls the apex downward	Hypoglossal nerve (cranial nerve XII)
Transverse	Median fibrous septum	Fibrous tissues at lateral margins	Makes the tongue narrower and elongates it	Hypoglossal nerve (cranial nerve XII)
Vertical	Mucous membrane of tongue dorsum	Inferior and lateral tongue margins	Flattens and widens the tongue	Hypoglossal nerve (cranial nerve XII)
Extrinsic Tongue Muscles				
Palatoglossus (forms palatoglossal arc or anterior faucial pillars)	Inferior surface of palatine aponeurosis	Transverse and posterolateral muscular portions of the tongue	Lifts the tongue and pulls it backward Constricts the posterior limits of the oral cavity (to isolate from oropharynx)	Pharyngeal branch of the vagus nerve (cranial nerve X) via the pharyngeal plexus
Styloglossus	Styloid process of the temporal bone Stylomandibular ligament	Posterolateral portion of the tongue	Lifts the sides of the tongue Retracts the base of the tongue	Hypoglossal nerve (cranial nerve XII)
Hyoglossus	Greater horn and body of hyoid	Lateral sides of the tongue	Pulls down the sides of the tongue	Hypoglossal nerve (cranial nerve XII)
Genioglossus	Superior mental spine (genial tubercle) on the internal surface of the mandible	Back and apex of the tongue Inferior fibers insert on the hyoid bone	Protrudes the tongue and depresses central portion Also has been reported that a unilateral contraction moves the tongue on opposite side	Hypoglossal nerve (cranial nerve XII)

Muscles of Mastication (see Figures 3.15 [p. 135] and 3.20 [p. 147])

Muscles	Origin	Insertion	Action(s)	Innervation
Jaw-Closing Muscles				
Masseter (superficial and deep)	Zygomatic process of the maxilla Zygomatic arch	External surface of the angle and ramus of the mandible Coronoid process of the mandible	Elevates the mandible Superficial: helps protrude the mandible Deep: contributes to retraction of the mandible	Masseter nerve of the mandibular division of the trigeminal nerve (cranial nerve V)
Temporalis (anterior, middle, and posterior portions)	Temporal fossa	Coronoid process of the mandible Anterior surface of the ramus of the mandible	Contraction of anterior and middle fibers elevates mandible Contraction of posterior fibers may elevate and retract mandible Unilateral contraction may contribute to lateral movement of mandible	Deep temporal nerve of the mandibular division of the trigeminal nerve (cranial nerve V)
Medial (internal) pterygoid	Medial surface of lateral pterygoid plate of sphenoid Pyramidal process of the palatine bone Maxillary tuberosity	Internal surface of the angle and ramus of the mandible	Elevates the mandible with temporalis and masseter muscles Protrudes mandible with lateral pterygoid and masseter muscles Unilateral contracting: moves jaw laterally (opposite side)	Medial pterygoid nerve of the mandibular division of the trigeminal nerve (cranial nerve V)
Jaw-Opening Muscles				
Lateral (external) pterygoid	Superior: greater wing of sphenoid Inferior: external surface of lateral pterygoid plate of sphenoid	Articular disc of the temporomandibular joint Condylar process of the mandible	Superior: co-activated with jaw-closing muscles Inferior: bilateral contraction protrudes mandible Unilateral contraction: moves mandible laterally toward the opposite side (grinding)	Anterior trunk of mandibular division of the trigeminal nerve (cranial nerve V)
Digastric	Medial surface of the mastoid process of temporal bone	Lower border of the mandible near the midline with the intermediate tendon tethered to the hyoid by a fibrous loop of connective tissue	With the mandible stabilized, aids in elevating the hyoid bone, which is necessary for swallowing Opens jaw when the hyoid bone is fixed	Posterior belly: digastric branch of the facial nerve (cranial nerve VII) Anterior belly: mylohyoid branch of the inferior alveolar nerve of the mandibular division of the trigeminal nerve (cranial nerve V)
Mylohyoid	Mylohyoid line (internal oblique line) of the internal surface of the mandible	Anterior and middle fibers: midline raphe, where fibers are linked with those of the opposite side Posterior fibers: body of the hyoid bone	Elevates the floor of the mouth and the hyoid bone Contributes to jaw opening if hyoid bone is fixed	Mylohyoid branch of the inferior alveolar nerve of the mandibular division of the trigeminal nerve (cranial nerve V)
Geniohyoid	Inferior mental spine on the internal surface of the mandible	Anterior surface of the body of the hyoid bone	Contributes to jaw opening if hyoid bone is fixed	First cervical spinal nerve (C1) traveling with fibers of the hypoglossal nerve (cranial nerve XII)

Muscles of the Soft Palate (see Figure 3.23 [p. 153])

Muscles	Origin	Insertion	Action(s)	Innervation
Levator veli palatini	Petrous portion of temporal bone Inferior aspect of the cartilaginous pharyngotympanic tube	Palatine raphe (aponeurosis)	Elevates the soft palate and may contribute to dilate pharyngotympanic tube	Pharyngeal branch of the vagus nerve (cranial nerve X) via the pharyngeal plexus
Tensor veli palatini	Scaphoid fossa Spine of the sphenoid Lateral cartilaginous walls of the pharyngotympanic tube	The tendon wraps around the pterygoid hamulus and inserts into the palatine aponeurosis and the horizontal plates of the palatine bone	Dilates the pharyngotympanic tube during swallowing and yawning and tenses the palate	Medial pterygoid nerve of mandibular division of the trigeminal nerve (cranial nerve V)
Palatoglossus (forms palatoglossal arch or anterior faucial pillars)	Inferior surface of the palatine aponeurosis	Transverse and posterolateral muscular portions of the tongue	Lifts the tongue and pulls it backward Constricts the posterior limits of the oral cavity (to isolate from oropharynx)	Pharyngeal branch of the vagus nerve (cranial nerve X) via the pharyngeal plexus
Palatopharyngeus (forms palatopharyngeal arch or posterior faucial pillars)	Palatine aponeurosis	Posterior border of thyroid cartilage Inferior portion of pharynx	Pulls the soft palate down Constricts and lifts the pharynx Helps direct the bolus into the pharynx during swallowing	Pharyngeal branch of the vagus nerve (cranial nerve X) via the pharyngeal plexus
Uvular	Posterior nasal spine Palatine aponeurosis	Mucosa of the uvula	May play a role in elevation of the soft palate	Pharyngeal branch of the vagus nerve (cranial nerve X) via the pharyngeal plexus

Muscles of the Pharynx (see Figure 3.24 [p. 156])

Muscles	Origin	Insertion	Action(s)	Innervation
Superior pharyngeal constrictor	Medial pterygoid plate, pterygomandibular raphe, and mylohyoid line of mandible	Median pharyngeal raphe Pharyngeal tubercle on the basilar part of occipital bone	Reduces pharyngeal diameter during swallowing (propulsive pressure acting on bolus) and assists in velopharyngeal closure	Pharyngeal branch of the vagus nerve (cranial nerve X) via the pharyngeal plexus
Middle pharyngeal constrictor	Great horns of the hyoid bone and stylohyoid ligament	Median pharyngeal raphe	Reduces pharyngeal diameter during swallowing (propulsive pressure acting on bolus)	Pharyngeal branch of the vagus nerve (cranial nerve X) via the pharyngeal plexus
Inferior pharyngeal constrictor	Most fibers originate from thyroid lamina (thyropharyngeus muscle) Some originate from cricoid cartilage (cricopharyngeus muscle)	Median pharyngeal raphe (with the exception of the fibers that form the cricopharyngeus)	Reduces the diameter of the inferior portions of the pharynx (thyropharyngeus muscle) Acts as the sphincter-like opening to the cervical esophagus during swallowing (cricopharyngeus muscle)	Pharyngeal branch of the vagus nerve (cranial nerve X) via the pharyngeal plexus, in addition to recurrent laryngeal nerve and external branch of the superior laryngeal nerve of the vagus nerve (cranial nerve X)
Salpingopharyngeus muscle	Inferoposterior surface of the cartilage of the pharyngotympanic tube	Lateral walls of the pharynx (fibers mix with palatopharyngeus)	Contributes to elevation of the pharynx during swallowing and may contribute to the distortion of the tubal cartilage of the pharyngotympanic tube to permit aeration of the middle ear	Pharyngeal branch of the vagus (cranial nerve X) via the pharyngeal plexus
Stylopharyngeus muscle	Base of the styloid process of the temporal bone	Mucous membrane of the pharynx and on the thyroid cartilage	Elevates the larynx and elevates and expands the pharynx during swallowing	Glossopharyngeal nerve (cranial nerve IX)

AUDITORY SYSTEM

■ OVERVIEW

Hearing is vital to spoken language perception and production. Hearing impairment can drastically affect speech and language development in the infant and child. In the adult, hearing is an extremely important feedback source for appropriate speech sound production. It is also extremely important for many other aspects of day-to-day living, including the perception of music and other environmental sounds. Hearing is thus a crucial function that affects many aspects of quality of life in addition to its role in speech and language.

The study of the anatomy (structures) and function of the peripheral hearing system is typically divided into three functional components: (1) the outer ear, (2) the middle ear, and (3) the inner ear. Each of these components serves a different but complementary role in the transduction of environmental acoustic vibrations into neural impulses (sound). The inner ear also contains the vestibular system that functions for balance and body orientation.

The role of the external or outer ear is to capture sounds and direct them to a membrane that converts acoustic vibrations to mechanical energy. The membrane and three attached small bones and supporting muscles and ligaments in the middle ear transmit these sounds to the sensory end organ of hearing in the inner ear (cochlea). They also provide an important impedance matching function between airborne sounds in the environment and fluid vibrations in the cochlea. In the cochlea, differences in stiffness along the basilar membrane cause it to vibrate with the greatest amplitude at different places along its length for different frequencies of sound. This stimulates complex and delicate sensory receptors, which transduce the motion into neural activity in the auditory nerve and higher levels of the central auditory system.

This chapter covers the vestibular system and the three functional components of the peripheral hearing system—the outer ear, middle ear, and inner ear—and the central auditory pathway.

■ ANATOMICAL DIVISIONS OF THE EAR

The ear is divided into the following three major sections (Figure 4.1):

1. The outer ear is composed of the auricle and external acoustic meatus.
2. The middle ear is composed of the tympanic cavity, the middle ear ossicles (the *malleus*, the *incus*, and the *stapes*), and the middle ear muscles.
3. The inner ear is composed of the osseous and membranous labyrinths.

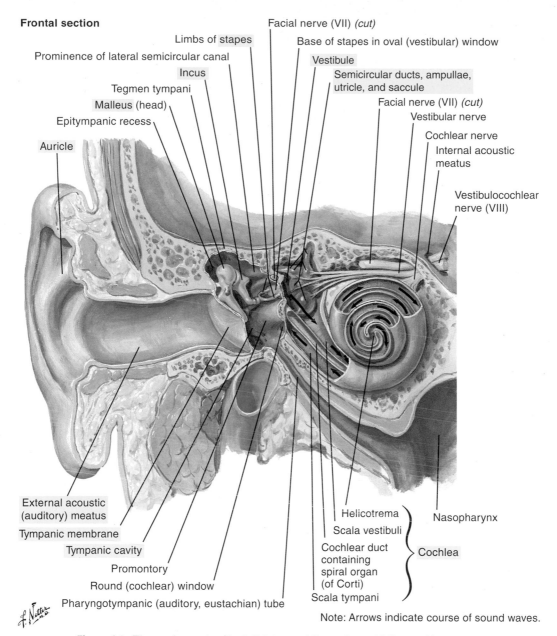

Frontal section

Limbs of stapes
Prominence of lateral semicircular canal
Incus
Tegmen tympani
Malleus (head)
Epitympanic recess
Auricle

Facial nerve (VII) *(cut)*
Base of stapes in oval (vestibular) window
Vestibule
Semicircular ducts, ampullae, utricle, and saccule
Facial nerve (VII) *(cut)*
Vestibular nerve
Cochlear nerve
Internal acoustic meatus
Vestibulocochlear nerve (VIII)

External acoustic (auditory) meatus
Tympanic membrane
Tympanic cavity
Promontory
Round (cochlear) window
Pharyngotympanic (auditory, eustachian) tube

Helicotrema
Scala vestibuli
Cochlear duct containing spiral organ (of Corti)
Scala tympani

Nasopharynx

Cochlea

Note: Arrows indicate course of sound waves.

Figure 4.1. The main anatomical divisions of the outer, middle, and inner ear.

Note Labels of certain figures are highlighted in yellow to emphasize the related elements in the corresponding text.

■ OUTER EAR

Auricle or Pinna (Figure 4.2; see also Figure 4.1 [p. 177])

The auricle, or pinna, is a flaplike structure that helps direct sound waves into the external acoustic meatus and aids in sound localization. Some animals can move their pinna extensively for additional directional selectivity. It is composed of fibrocartilage covered by skin and attached to the temporal bone by several extrinsic muscles and ligaments. Internal ligaments and muscles join auricular structures. The following are prominent surface landmarks:

- The helix is the curved outer rim.
- The crus of the helix divides the concha into two parts, with the inferior portion being the entrance to the external acoustic meatus.
- The auricular tubercle (of Darwin) is a small projection sometimes found on the lateral border of the helix.
- The antihelix is a second semicircular ridge anterior to the helix.
- The triangular fossa lies between the two crura of the antihelix.
- The scaphoid fossa lies between the helix and the antihelix.
- The tragus is the flap partially covering the entrance to the external acoustic meatus.
- The antitragus is the smaller flap opposite the tragus.
- The lobule of the auricle (earlobe) is the noncartilaginous and highly vascular inferior extremity.

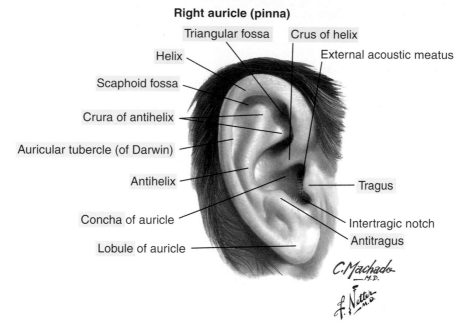

Figure 4.2. The auricle, or pinna.

External Acoustic (Auditory) Meatus or Ear Canal (see Figure 4.1 [p. 177])

The external acoustic meatus, or ear canal, is an oval, S-shaped tube approximately 25 to 35 mm long and approximately 6 to 8 mm in diameter. The lateral third is cartilage and continuous with the cartilage of the auricle. The medial two-thirds are osseous. It contains cilia and glands that produce wax (ceruminous glands) and oils (sebaceous glands), and these keep the external acoustic meatus clean and supple. These substances also help, in combination with the shape of the tube, to prevent foreign bodies (such as insects) from entering the meatus. The resonating frequencies of the meatus are such that sensitivity is increased to sounds between approximately 1000 and 6000 Hz.

Tympanic Membrane, Tympanum, or Eardrum (Figure 4.3)

The tympanic membrane is a very thin but resilient membrane that vibrates in response to acoustic energy. It sits obliquely at the end of the external acoustic meatus. It is approximately 10 mm in diameter, and its shape is almost circular; its thickened outer ring (annulus) attaches to a groove in the tympanic cavity (tympanic sulcus). The normal appearance of the tympanic membrane (e.g., during visual inspection with an otoscope) is concave, smooth, and translucent. When illuminated, an important landmark, the "cone of light," can normally be seen radiating from a central depression whose deepest point, called the *umbo,* is formed by the attachment of the manubrium of the malleus (a middle ear ossicle). The process of the malleus can be seen extending toward the superior border.

The tympanic membrane has the following three layers:

1. The outer cutaneous layer is a thin layer continuous with the lining of the external acoustic meatus.
2. The middle fibrous layer is more substantial and composed of circular and radial fibers. It is deficient at the superior border, which creates the pars flaccida. The rest of the membrane is the pars tensa.
3. The internal mucous layer is continuous with the lining of the tympanic cavity.

Coronal oblique section of external acoustic meatus and middle ear (tympanic cavity)

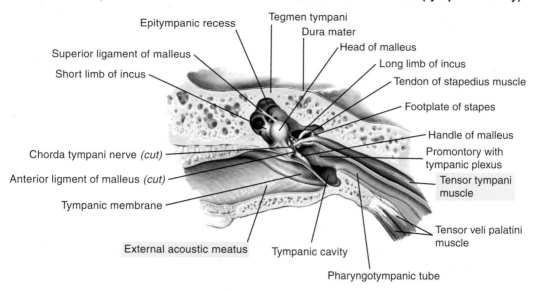

Epitympanic recess

Superior ligament of malleus

Short limb of incus

Tegmen tympani

Dura mater

Head of malleus

Long limb of incus

Tendon of stapedius muscle

Footplate of stapes

Handle of malleus

Promontory with tympanic plexus

Tensor tympani muscle

Chorda tympani nerve *(cut)*

Anterior ligament of malleus *(cut)*

Tympanic membrane

External acoustic meatus

Tympanic cavity

Tensor veli palatini muscle

Pharyngotympanic tube

Otoscopic view of right tympanic membrane

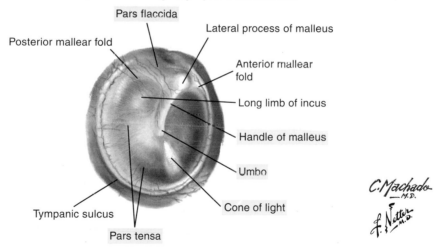

Pars flaccida

Posterior mallear fold

Lateral process of malleus

Anterior mallear fold

Long limb of incus

Handle of malleus

Umbo

Cone of light

Tympanic sulcus

Pars tensa

C. Machado M.D.

F. Netter M.D.

Figure 4.3. The external acoustic (auditory) meatus *(top)* and tympanic membrane *(bottom)*.

■ MIDDLE EAR

Tympanic Cavity or Middle Ear Cavity (Figure 4.4; see also Figures 4.1 [p. 177] and 4.3 [p. 181])

A roughly rectangular air-filled cavity ("box"), the tympanic cavity lies medial to the tympanic membrane within the petrous portion of the temporal bone. It is formed by two cavities: (1) the epitympanic recess and (2) the tympanic cavity proper.

Epitympanic Recess

The epitympanic recess is superior to the tympanic membrane. It contains the head of the malleus and most of the incus.

Tympanic Cavity Proper

The tympanic cavity proper is the "box" containing the middle ear ossicular system and points of communication with the inner ear and pharyngotympanic tube. The tegmental (superior) wall, or roof, is a thin plate of bone separating the tympanic cavity from the cranium and is called the *tegmen tympani*. The jugular (inferior) wall, or floor, is a thin bone that separates the tympanic cavity from the internal jugular vein. The tympanic nerve, a branch of the glossopharyngeal nerve (cranial nerve IX), passes through the floor of the tympanic cavity.

The membranous (lateral) wall is the tympanic membrane. The labyrinthine (medial) walls are the oval window (fenestra vestibule) and, below, the round window (fenestra rotunda). Superior to the oval window passes the chorda tympani nerve (a branch of the facial [VII] cranial nerve). The carotid (anterior) wall separates the tympanic cavity from the carotid artery. Superiorly, a canal houses the tensor tympani muscle and, more inferiorly, the opening of the pharyngotympanic tube connects the tympanic cavity to the nasopharynx (see later).

The mastoid (posterior) wall on the posterosuperior border is the mastoid antrum, a sinus with several openings to the mastoid air cells. It provides a path of direct communication between air cells and the tympanic cavity, in addition to a potential path for the life-threatening infection mastoiditis. Inferior to this is the pyramidal eminence, the point of emergence of the tendon of the stapedial muscle. Lateral to this is the chordal eminence, the point of emergence of the chorda tympani nerve into the tympanic cavity.

Lateral wall of tympanic cavity: medial (internal) view

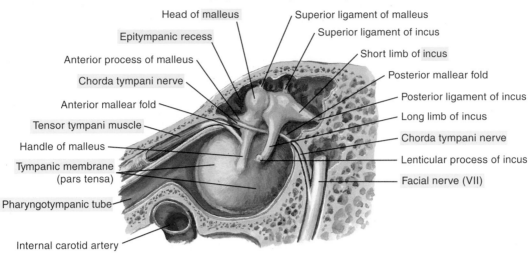

Head of malleus
Epitympanic recess
Anterior process of malleus
Chorda tympani nerve
Anterior mallear fold
Tensor tympani muscle
Handle of malleus
Tympanic membrane (pars tensa)
Pharyngotympanic tube
Internal carotid artery

Superior ligament of malleus
Superior ligament of incus
Short limb of incus
Posterior mallear fold
Posterior ligament of incus
Long limb of incus
Chorda tympani nerve
Lenticular process of incus
Facial nerve (VII)

Medial wall of tympanic cavity: lateral view

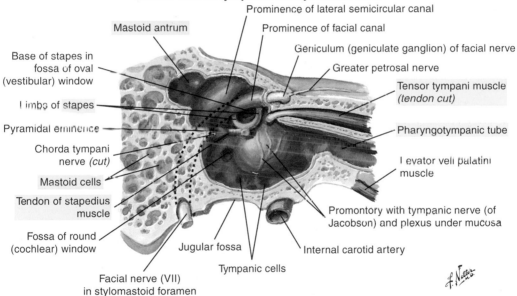

Prominence of lateral semicircular canal
Mastoid antrum
Prominence of facial canal
Geniculum (geniculate ganglion) of facial nerve
Greater petrosal nerve
Base of stapes in fossa of oval (vestibular) window
Limbs of stapes
Pyramidal eminence
Chorda tympani nerve (cut)
Mastoid cells
Tendon of stapedius muscle
Fossa of round (cochlear) window
Tensor tympani muscle (tendon cut)
Pharyngotympanic tube
Levator veli palatini muscle
Promontory with tympanic nerve (of Jacobson) and plexus under mucosa
Jugular fossa
Tympanic cells
Internal carotid artery
Facial nerve (VII) in stylomastoid foramen

Figure 4.4. The tympanic cavity.

Middle Ear Ossicles (Figure 4.5; see also Figure 4.4 [p. 183])

The tympanic cavity proper houses the middle ear ossicles and their supporting ligaments and muscles. This system transmits acoustic vibrations from the tympanic membrane to the inner ear. Cartilaginous synovial joints connect the three ossicles.

Malleus ("Hammer")

The malleus, or "hammer," is the largest (but still only 9 mm long) and most lateral of the middle ear ossicles. It is suspended in the tympanic cavity by three ligaments; the most significant is the anterior ligament of the malleus. The manubrium (handle) is attached to the tympanic membrane. The tendon of the tensor tympani muscle (see later) attaches to the upper portion of the manubrium.

Incus ("Anvil")

The incus, or "anvil," articulates medially with the malleus and through an inferior projection (which terminates in the lenticular process) with the stapes. It is suspended from the tympanic cavity by the posterior ligament of the incus.

Stapes ("Stirrup")

The stapes, or "stirrup," is the smallest bone in the human body. Its footplate attaches to the oval window of the cochlea by the annular ligament. The tendon of the stapedial muscle is attached to the neck of the stapes.

Middle Ear Muscles (see Figure 4.3 [p. 181] and 4.4 [p. 183])

Tensor Tympani

The tensor tympani is a muscle contained within a bony canal above and running along the pharyngotympanic tube. Its tendon enters the tympanic cavity and attaches to the manubrium of the malleus near the tympanic membrane.

The tensor tympani is innervated by a branch of the mandibular division of the trigeminal nerve (cranial nerve V).

Stapedial Muscle or Stapedius

The stapedius is the smallest striated muscle in the body. Its tendon emerges from the pyramidal eminence to insert on the posterior surface of the neck of the stapes.

The stapedial muscle is innervated by the nerve to the stapedius of the facial nerve (cranial nerve VII).

Action of the Middle Ear Muscles

Muscular contraction increases the stiffness of the ossicular chain. Reflex activation may provide some sound protection benefits against intense, low-frequency sounds (below 1 to 2 kHz). Protection against rapid-onset sounds is minimal because of reflex delays (approximately 60 to 120 ms). Activation may reduce sensitivity to self-generated vocalizations transmitted to the cochlea via bone conduction.

The acoustic reflex (AR) activation of the middle ear muscles is a diagnostic tool used in the practice of audiology to assess the function of the middle ear and higher-order neural processes involved in hearing.

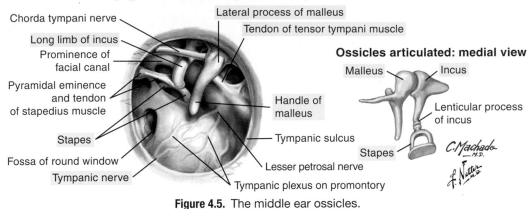

Figure 4.5. The middle ear ossicles.

Pharyngotympanic (Auditory, Eustachian) Tube (Figure 4.6; see also Figure 4.4 [p. 183])

The pharyngotympanic tube is approximately 35 to 38 mm long and extends downward, forward, and medially from the tympanic cavity to the nasopharynx. The lateral portion is osseous, and the medial portion is composed of cartilage and other connective tissue. The pharyngotympanic tube is normally closed by elastic recoil forces (and potentially by tension provided by muscles such as the salpingopharyngeus) to protect the middle ear from pathogens.

The tube opens during swallowing and yawning, principally by action of the tensor veli palatini, with potential contributions from the levator veli palatini and tensor tympani muscles. It equalizes pressure between the middle ear and external atmospheric pressure and allows the tympanic membrane to operate efficiently in a variety of atmospheric pressures. This tube also drains the tympanic cavity and aerates tissues. The pharyngotympanic tube is shorter and more horizontally placed in children and thus provides a more direct path for middle ear infections such as otitis media.

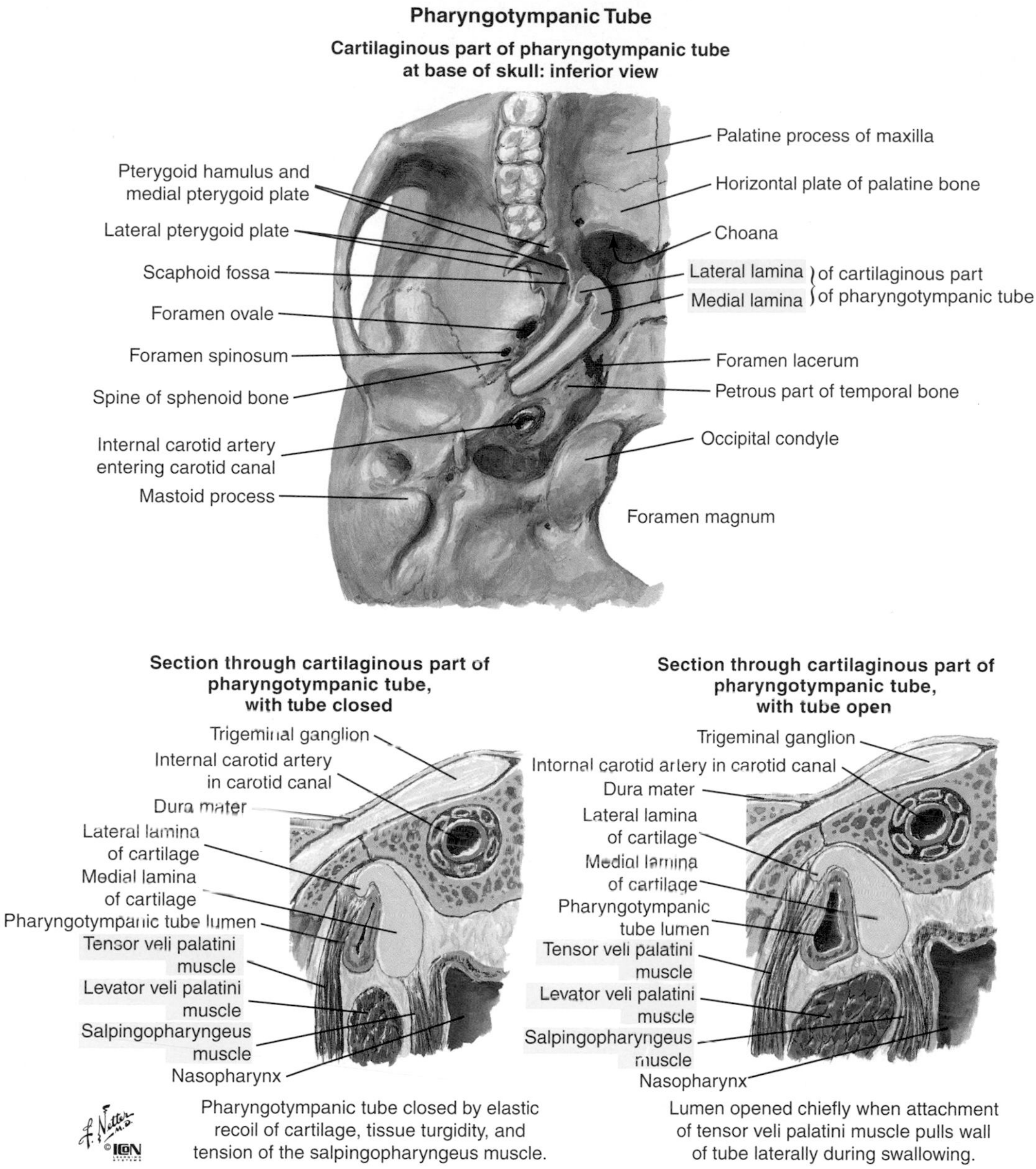

Pharyngotympanic Tube

**Cartilaginous part of pharyngotympanic tube
at base of skull: inferior view**

Pterygoid hamulus and
medial pterygoid plate

Lateral pterygoid plate

Scaphoid fossa

Foramen ovale

Foramen spinosum

Spine of sphenoid bone

Internal carotid artery
entering carotid canal

Mastoid process

Palatine process of maxilla

Horizontal plate of palatine bone

Choana

Lateral lamina ⟩ of cartilaginous part
Medial lamina ⟩ of pharyngotympanic tube

Foramen lacerum

Petrous part of temporal bone

Occipital condyle

Foramen magnum

**Section through cartilaginous part of
pharyngotympanic tube,
with tube closed**

Trigeminal ganglion

Internal carotid artery
in carotid canal

Dura mater

Lateral lamina
of cartilage

Medial lamina
of cartilage

Pharyngotympanic tube lumen

Tensor veli palatini
muscle

Levator veli palatini
muscle

Salpingopharyngeus
muscle

Nasopharynx

Pharyngotympanic tube closed by elastic
recoil of cartilage, tissue turgidity, and
tension of the salpingopharyngeus muscle.

**Section through cartilaginous part of
pharyngotympanic tube,
with tube open**

Trigeminal ganglion

Internal carotid artery in carotid canal

Dura mater

Lateral lamina
of cartilage

Medial lamina
of cartilage

Pharyngotympanic
tube lumen

Tensor veli palatini
muscle

Levator veli palatini
muscle

Salpingopharyngeus
muscle

Nasopharynx

Lumen opened chiefly when attachment
of tensor veli palatini muscle pulls wall
of tube laterally during swallowing.

Figure 4.6. The pharyngotympanic (auditory, eustachian) tube.

■ INNER EAR

The inner ear is composed of two labyrinthine ("mazelike") systems: (1) the bony (osseous) outer labyrinth and (2) the internal membranous labyrinth.

Osseous or Bony Labyrinth (Figures 4.7, 4.8 [p. 190], and 4.9 [p. 191]; see also Figure 4.1 [p. 177])

The bony labyrinth is composed of a series of ducts and cavities within the petrous portion of the temporal bone. It contains the vestibule, the semicircular canals, and the coiled cochlea and is composed of tissue denser than the surrounding temporal bone.

Semicircular Canals

The semicircular canals are the lateral-most portion of the bony labyrinth. Anterior, posterior, and lateral canals are oriented approximately orthogonally.

Vestibule

The vestibule is interposed between the cochlea and the semicircular canals. The oval window is the entrance to the cochlea and point of attachment of the footplate of the stapes.

Cochlea

The cochlea is the medial-most portion of the bony labyrinth. This cavity (also called the *spiral canal*) is approximately 35 mm long and coiled around a central core of bone called the *modiolus* for approximately 2¾ turns from the base (basal turn) to the apex. Small perforations in the modiolus and projecting shelf (osseous spiral lamina) allow passage of auditory nerve fibers that innervate the sensory end organs of hearing located in the membranous labyrinth (see Figures 4.11 [p. 194] and 4.12 [p. 197]).

The spiral canal of the osseous cochlea contains three channels: the middle cochlear duct (a component of the membranous labyrinth, see later), the scala vestibuli (above), and scala tympani (below) (see Figures 4.7, 4.11 [p. 194], and 4.12 [p. 197]). The scala vestibuli is the only channel within the osseous cochlea in direct contact with the vestibule (thus its name) and communicates with the scala tympani at the apex of the cochlea. A round window is located at the end of the scala tympani and has a membranous covering that provides a point of expansion for fluid movement within the cochlea. The cochlear duct contains endolymph, and the scala vestibuli and scala tympani contain perilymph.

Bony and membranous labyrinths

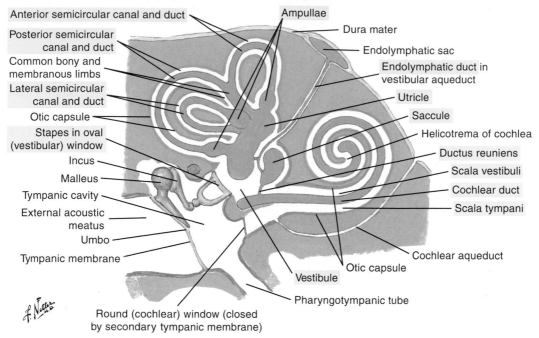

Anterior semicircular canal and duct
Posterior semicircular canal and duct
Common bony and membranous limbs
Lateral semicircular canal and duct
Otic capsule
Stapes in oval (vestibular) window
Incus
Malleus
Tympanic cavity
External acoustic meatus
Umbo
Tympanic membrane
Round (cochlear) window (closed by secondary tympanic membrane)
Ampullae
Dura mater
Endolymphatic sac
Endolymphatic duct in vestibular aqueduct
Utricle
Saccule
Helicotrema of cochlea
Ductus reuniens
Scala vestibuli
Cochlear duct
Scala tympani
Cochlear aqueduct
Otic capsule
Vestibule
Pharyngotympanic tube

Figure 4.7. Schema of the bony and membranous labyrinths of the inner ear.

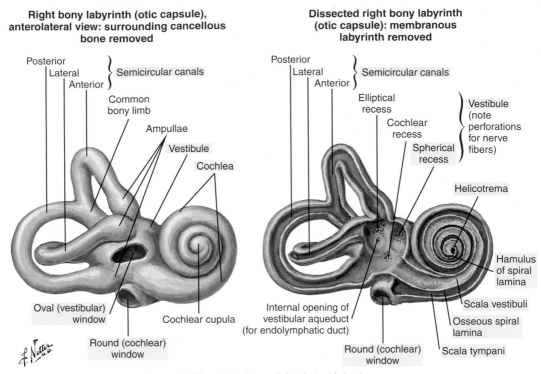

Figure 4.8. The right bony labyrinth of the inner ear.

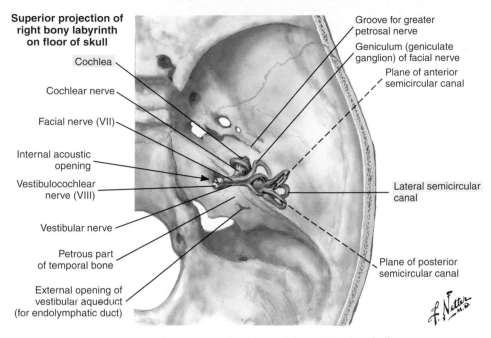

Superior projection of right bony labyrinth on floor of skull

Cochlea

Cochlear nerve

Facial nerve (VII)

Internal acoustic opening

Vestibulocochlear nerve (VIII)

Vestibular nerve

Petrous part of temporal bone

External opening of vestibular aqueduct (for endolymphatic duct)

Groove for greater petrosal nerve

Geniculum (geniculate ganglion) of facial nerve

Plane of anterior semicircular canal

Lateral semicircular canal

Plane of posterior semicircular canal

Figure 4.9. Orientation of the bony labyrinth in the skull.

Membranous Labyrinth (Figure 4.10)

The membranous labyrinth is suspended within the osseous labyrinth and contains the sensory end organs of hearing and balance. It is filled with a fluid called *endolymph*. The membranous labyrinth can be divided into two functional regions: the vestibular and cochlear labyrinths. The sensory end organs of the vestibular labyrinth are involved in balance and body orientation, whereas the sensory end organs within the cochlear labyrinth are involved in hearing.

Vestibular Labyrinth (Figures 4.10 and 4.11 [p. 194]; see also Figure 4.7 [p. 189])

The vestibular labyrinth is made up of three membranous semicircular ducts and two otolithic organs.

Semicircular Ducts

Three semicircular membranous ducts occupy approximately one-quarter of the diameter of their own osseous semicircular canals. They communicate with the utricle. Each of the ducts widens at their lateral ends to form ampullae. Part of the membranous wall of each ampulla is slightly elevated and forms an important vestibular receptor called the *ampullary crest* that contains sensory (hair) cells sensitive to head rotation. The stereocilia (ciliated tops of the hair cells) that can be found on each hair cell are embedded into a gelatinous mass that occupies a major portion of the ampullae called the *cupula* (see Figure 4.11 [p. 194]).

Otolithic Organs

The otolithic organs are two membranous sacs located in the vestibule, the utricle, and the saccule. The utricle is bigger and lies in the posterosuperior region of the vestibule. The smaller saccule is located in the spherical recess of the vestibule. The utricle and saccule communicate via the utriculosaccular duct (which gives rise to the endolymphatic duct). The saccule also communicates with the cochlear duct via the ductus reuniens. Part of the epithelium lining the internal wall of the otolithic organs contains specialized sensory epithelia that form important vestibular receptors, the maculae. These specialized sensory epithelia contain hair cells that are sensitive to movements of the head in the vertical and horizontal planes. The stereocilia that can be found on the top of each hair cell are embedded into a gelatinous otolithic membrane covered by small crystals of calcium carbonate called *otoconia* (otoliths, statoliths) (see Figure 4.11 [p. 194]). In the anatomical position, the utricular maculae are oriented horizontally, whereas the saccular maculae are oriented vertically.

Right membranous labyrinth with nerves: posteromedial view

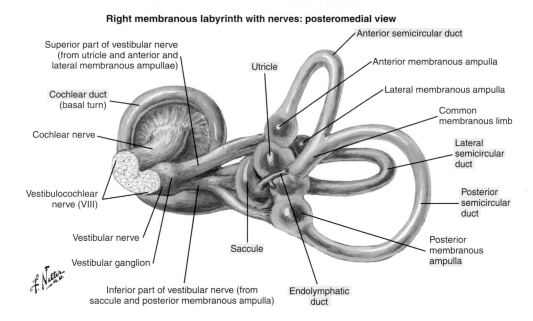

Superior part of vestibular nerve
(from utricle and anterior and
lateral membranous ampullae)

Cochlear duct
(basal turn)

Cochlear nerve

Vestibulocochlear
nerve (VIII)

Vestibular nerve

Vestibular ganglion

Inferior part of vestibular nerve (from
saccule and posterior membranous ampulla)

Utricle

Anterior semicircular duct

Anterior membranous ampulla

Lateral membranous ampulla

Common
membranous limb

Lateral
semicircular
duct

Posterior
semicircular
duct

Posterior
membranous
ampulla

Saccule

Endolymphatic
duct

Lateral projection of right membranous labyrinth

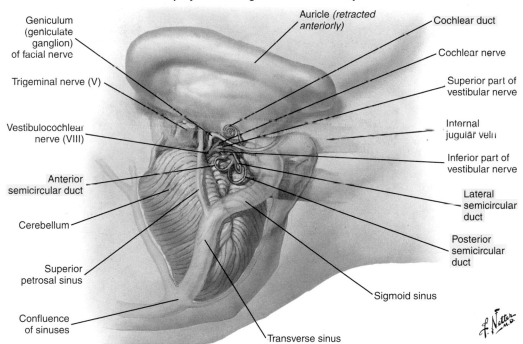

Geniculum
(geniculate
ganglion)
of facial nerve

Trigeminal nerve (V)

Vestibulocochlear
nerve (VIII)

Anterior
semicircular duct

Cerebellum

Superior
petrosal sinus

Confluence
of sinuses

Auricle (retracted
anteriorly)

Cochlear duct

Cochlear nerve

Superior part of
vestibular nerve

Internal
jugular vein

Inferior part of
vestibular nerve

Lateral
semicircular
duct

Posterior
semicircular
duct

Sigmoid sinus

Transverse sinus

Figure 4.10. The membranous labyrinth of the inner ear and its orientation in the skull.

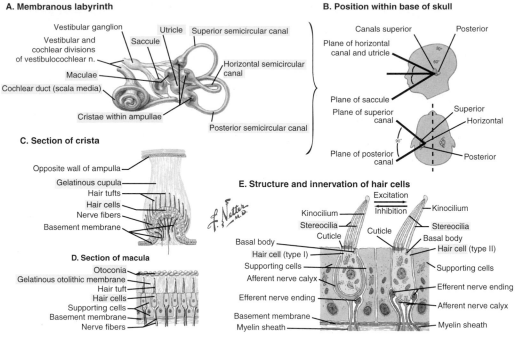

A. Membranous labyrinth

Vestibular ganglion

Vestibular and cochlear divisions of vestibulocochlear n.

Maculae

Cochlear duct (scala media)

Cristae within ampullae

Saccule

Utricle   Superior semicircular canal

Horizontal semicircular canal

Posterior semicircular canal

B. Position within base of skull

Canals superior   Posterior

Plane of horizontal canal and utricle

30°
60°

Plane of saccule

Plane of superior canal

Plane of posterior canal

90°

Superior

Horizontal

Posterior

C. Section of crista

Opposite wall of ampulla

Gelatinous cupula

Hair tufts

Hair cells

Nerve fibers

Basement membrane

F. Netter m.d.

E. Structure and innervation of hair cells

Excitation

Inhibition

Kinocilium

Stereocilia

Cuticle

Basal body

Hair cell (type I)

Supporting cells

Afferent nerve calyx

Efferent nerve ending

Basement membrane

Myelin sheath

Kinocilium

Stereocilia

Basal body

Hair cell (type II)

Supporting cells

Efferent nerve ending

Afferent nerve calyx

Myelin sheath

Cuticle

D. Section of macula

Otoconia

Gelatinous otolithic membrane

Hair tuft

Hair cells

Supporting cells

Basement membrane

Nerve fibers

Figure 4.11. Vestibular receptors.

Cochlear Labyrinth

Cochlear Duct or Scala Media (see Figures 4.12 [p. 197]; see also Figures 4.7 [p. 189] and 4.10 [p. 193])
The cochlear labyrinth consists of the cochlear duct (scala media), which is a spirally arranged tube approximately 33 mm long and suspended within the spiral canal of the osseous cochlea. The superior and inferior bounds of the cochlear duct are formed, respectively, by the Reissner's membrane and the basilar membrane. The cochlear duct contains the sensory end organ of hearing, the organ of Corti.

Reissner's Membrane (see Figures 4.12 [p. 197] and 4.13 [p. 198])
The Reissner's membrane extends obliquely above the basilar membrane from the osseous spiral lamina to the outer wall of the osseous cochlea. It joins the basilar membrane at the helicotrema at the apex of the cochlea. This membrane divides the scala vestibuli from the cochlear duct.

Basilar Membrane (see Figures 4.12 [p. 197] and 4.13 [p. 198])
The basilar membrane projects from the osseous spiral lamina and connects with the outer wall of the osseous cochlea via the spiral ligament. It divides the cochlear duct from scala tympani. Although the cross-sectional area of the bony labyrinth, or canal, becomes smaller as the apex is reached, the basilar membrane becomes wider. Thus the basilar membrane is wider and more flaccid at the apical end and narrower and stiffer at the base, and this influences its resonant properties and frequency-response characteristics. Sitting on the basilar membrane is the organ of Corti, which contains hair cells (sensory cells) and supporting cells.

Organ of Corti (Figures 4.12 and 4.13 [p. 198])

The organ of Corti contains sensory (hair) cells and supporting cells.

Inner Hair Cells. One row of approximately 3500 hair cells lies along the length of the cochlea on the inner side of the tunnel of Corti. Approximately 40 stereocilia (ciliated tops of the hair cells) on each cell are arranged in parallel rows of decreasing height toward the modiolus.

Outer Hair Cells. Three to five rows of approximately 12,000 cells are present. Approximately 150 stereocilia per hair cell are arranged in the form of a V or W, with the base of the letter pointing toward the spiral ligament and with decreasing height toward the modiolus side.

Tectorial Membrane. The tectorial membrane is semitransparent and gelatinous-like. Tips of the tallest row of outer hair cell stereocilia are in contact with the tectorial membrane, which extends over hair cells from the spiral limbus.

Supporting Cells. Hair cells and their stereocilia are held in place by several supporting cells, including the inner and outer pillars or rods of Corti (forming the inner tunnel of Corti) and the inner and outer phalangeal cells. A delicate reticular lamina holds the tops of the hair cells in place and allows for shearing forces on the stereocilia by the tectorial membrane.

Section through turn of cochlea

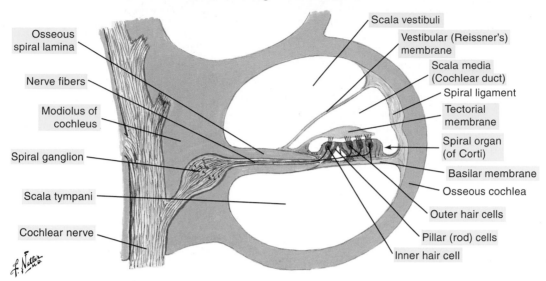

Osseous
spiral lamina

Nerve fibers

Modiolus of
cochleus

Spiral ganglion

Scala tympani

Cochlear nerve

Scala vestibuli

Vestibular (Reissner's)
membrane

Scala media
(Cochlear duct)

Spiral ligament

Tectorial
membrane

Spiral organ
(of Corti)

Basilar membrane

Osseous cochlea

Outer hair cells

Pillar (rod) cells

Inner hair cell

Figure 4.12. Cross-section through a turn of the cochlea.

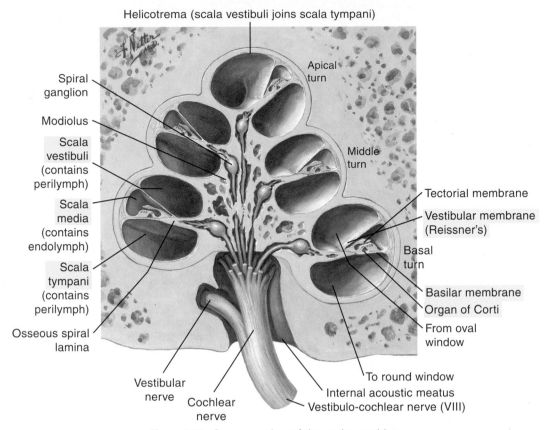

Figure 4.13. Cross-section of the entire cochlea.

■ COCHLEAR AFFERENT AND EFFERENT INNERVATION

Afferent Innervation

The cochlea is innervated by more than 30,000 sensory neurons. These afferent fibers of the eighth cranial nerve convey information from the cochlea to the central nervous system. Bipolar cells have their cell bodies in the spiral ganglion in the modiolus and send one process to synapse on the hair cells and a longer process (axon) to the cochlear nuclei. The process innervating the hair cells passes underneath the cells through openings in the spiral lamina called *habenula perforata*. There are two types of cochlear afferent fibers, as follows:
1. Inner radial, or type I, fibers
2. Outer spiral, or type II, fibers

Inner Radial, or Type I, Fibers

The inner radial, or type I, fibers represent 90% to 95% of all afferent fibers and innervate the inner hair cells exclusively. Each inner radial fiber goes to 1 inner hair cell, but each inner hair cell receives approximately 20 inner radial fibers; this is referred to as *many-to-one innervation*. These fibers are called *radial fibers* because they fan out in a radial direction.

Outer Spiral, or Type II, Fibers

The outer spiral, or type II, fibers cross the inner tunnel of Corti and "spiral" (run longitudinally) to synapse on multiple outer hair cells. One outer spiral fiber goes to many (approximately 10) outer hair cells *(one-to-many innervation)*.

Afferent Central Auditory Pathway (Figures 4.14 and 4.15 [p. 202])

Afferent nerve fibers (axons) carrying sensory information from the cochlea and the semi-circular canals together form the vestibulocochlear (or auditory) nerve (cranial nerve VIII). This nerve travels through the internal acoustic meatus to enter the brainstem at the junction of the pons and medulla. Auditory nerve fibers from the cochlea first synapse onto their respective cochlear nuclei (dorsal or ventral) located at the pontomedullary junction. These are referred to as *primary* or *first-order fibers.*

Beyond this lies the central auditory pathway. Fiber pathways or tracts made up of communicating axons from each ear travel ipsilaterally (on the same side) and contralaterally (on the opposite side) to higher levels of the nervous system, thus ensuring a redundancy of auditory information in the event of disease or damage.

Along the way, auditory sensory information is relayed or processed by a series of brainstem nuclei (collections of nerve cell bodies). The auditory brainstem nuclei include the superior olivary complex (in the pons), the lateral lemniscus (in the pons), the inferior colliculus (in the midbrain), and the medial geniculate body or nucleus (thalamic auditory relay nuclei). From there, fibers are distributed (auditory radiations) to the primary auditory cortex located on the transverse temporal gyrus (Heschl's gyrus) on the superior surface of the temporal lobe of each hemisphere.

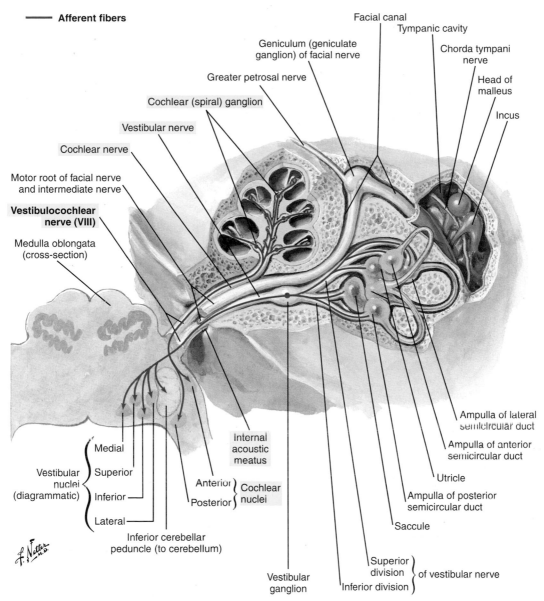

—— Afferent fibers

Facial canal

Geniculum (geniculate ganglion) of facial nerve

Tympanic cavity

Chorda tympani nerve

Greater petrosal nerve

Head of malleus

Cochlear (spiral) ganglion

Incus

Vestibular nerve

Cochlear nerve

Motor root of facial nerve and intermediate nerve

Vestibulocochlear nerve (VIII)

Medulla oblongata (cross-section)

Ampulla of lateral semicircular duct

Ampulla of anterior semicircular duct

Internal acoustic meatus

Utricle

Medial

Ampulla of posterior semicircular duct

Vestibular nuclei (diagrammatic)

Superior

Anterior

Cochlear nuclei

Inferior

Posterior

Saccule

Lateral

Inferior cerebellar peduncle (to cerebellum)

Superior division

of vestibular nerve

Inferior division

Vestibular ganglion

Figure 4.14. The vestibulocochlear nerve (cranial nerve VIII).

Afferent Auditory Pathways

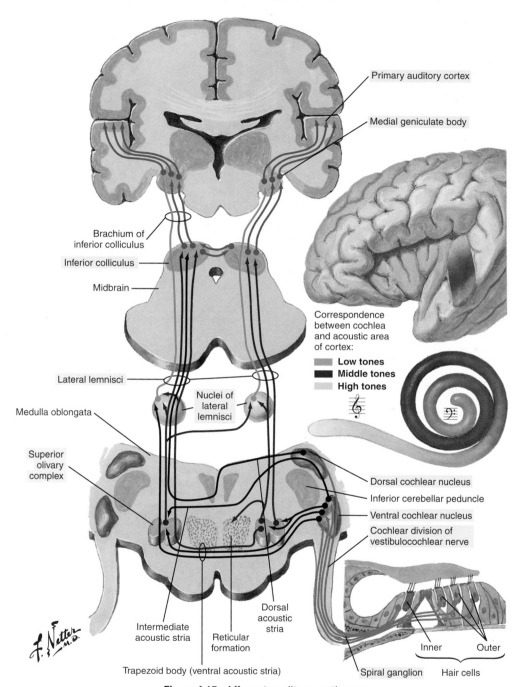

Primary auditory cortex

Medial geniculate body

Brachium of inferior colliculus

Inferior colliculus

Midbrain

Lateral lemnisci

Nuclei of lateral lemnisci

Medulla oblongata

Superior olivary complex

Correspondence between cochlea and acoustic area of cortex:

Low tones
Middle tones
High tones

Dorsal cochlear nucleus

Inferior cerebellar peduncle

Ventral cochlear nucleus

Cochlear division of vestibulocochlear nerve

Intermediate acoustic stria

Reticular formation

Dorsal acoustic stria

Trapezoid body (ventral acoustic stria)

Spiral ganglion

Hair cells

Inner   Outer

Figure 4.15. Afferent auditory pathways.

Efferent Central Auditory Pathway (Auditory Centrifugal Pathway)

A descending efferent pathway extends from the auditory cortex to the hair cells and interacts with the various processing stages (nuclei) of the ascending system, as previously described. The most well-understood part of the efferent pathway is the olivocochlear bundle, which runs from the superior olivary complex back to the hair cells in the cochlea. Medial olivocochlear bundle fibers innervate mainly outer hair cells and synapse directly on the base of the cell. This pathway may directly modulate the active process in the cochlea to sharpen perception and enhance auditory sensitivity to soft sounds. Lateral olivocochlear bundle fibers innervate primarily inner cells and synapse on the afferent fibers rather than directly on the cell. The action of this pathway is not yet well understood.

NERVOUS SYSTEM

◼ OVERVIEW

Speech production is an extremely complex sensorimotor behavior involving the coordinated action of numerous muscles distributed across several physiological systems, including the respiratory system, the laryngeal-phonatory system, and the oropharyngeal-articulatory system. Multiple control mechanisms are involved in the regulation of this complex system, including a higher-order motor control system, cognitive and linguistic components interacting with brainstem and cerebellum control systems, and a feedback-feedforward control system, which processes sensorimotor information arising from various sources.

Respiratory, laryngeal, and oropharyngeal structures are also involved in deglutition. Deglutition is important for both the transportation of food and saliva and the protection of the respiratory tract during wakefulness and sleep. Like speech production, deglutition is a complex behavior that involves several levels of neural control, including central pattern-generating circuitry interacting with sensory feedback and cortical control elements. Speech and deglutition appear to share common control elements.

The nervous system is divided into two parts: the central nervous system (brain and spinal cord) and the peripheral nervous system (spinal and cranial nerves). This chapter first examines the structures of the central nervous system and then examines the cranial and spinal nerves.

The brain develops from three primary structures: the rhombencephalon (or hindbrain), the mesencephalon (or midbrain), and the prosencephalon (or forebrain). The rhombencephalon in turn divides into the metencephalon (pons and cerebellum) and the myelencephalon (medulla). The prosencephalon divides into the telencephalon (cerebral hemispheres and basal ganglia) and the diencephalon (thalamus, hypothalamus, epithalamus, and subthalamus). The pons, medulla, and midbrain collectively form the *brainstem*.

**Developmental and Anatomical Divisions of the
Central Nervous System (CNS)**

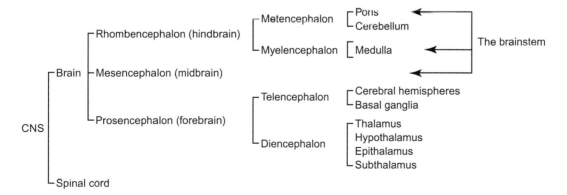

■ NEUROANATOMICAL TERMS OF DIRECTION (Figure 5.1)

When describing the location of structures in the brain, it is important to recognize that the neuroaxis flexes at the level of the midbrain during development. Thus when speaking of the upper portions of the brainstem (above the diencephalon) and the cerebral hemispheres, *rostral* (or anterior) refers to the front of the brain, and *caudal* (or posterior) refers to the back. *Dorsal* (or superior) is toward the top of the brain, and *ventral* (or inferior) is away from the top. Because of the superior-inferior orientation of the spinal cord and the lower portions of the brainstem, the terms of direction described in the introduction to this book apply.

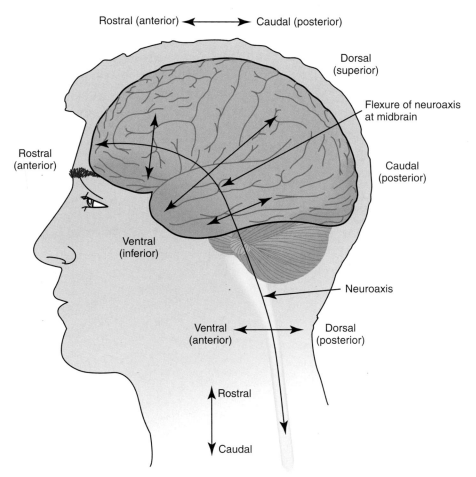

Figure 5.1. Neuroanatomical terms of direction.

■ TELENCEPHALON (CEREBRAL HEMISPHERES OR CEREBRUM AND BASAL GANGLIA) (Figures 5.2 [p. 212], 5.3 [p. 213], 5.4 [p. 214], 5.5 [p. 215], and 5.6 [p. 217])

Surface Structures

Characteristic Features

The telencephalon is composed of the two cerebral hemispheres separated by the longitudinal fissure (Figure 5.4 [p. 214]). Each hemisphere is composed of numerous irregular gyri (convolutions) separated by sulci (or fissures). The cerebral hemispheres are made up of gray matter (cell bodies) and white matter (nerve fiber axons). White matter fiber tracts are categorized as to whether they project to other brain areas (projection fibers), connect different areas within a cerebral hemisphere (association fibers), or join the two cerebral hemispheres (commissural fibers).

The cerebral cortex is the external, thin layer of gray matter capping the white matter core of the cerebral hemispheres. The cortex is stratified into six cellular layers (numbered from I to VI, starting from the most superficial layer). The laminar organization of the cortex into layers varies from region to region and reflects functional differences.

The organization of the cortical motor areas (i.e., the primary motor area, the supplementary motor area, and the lateral premotor cortex) is characterized by poor layering, such as the absence of layer IV, which contains granular cells, and the presence in layer V of giant pyramidal cells called *Betz cells*. The organization of the motor areas is referred to as *agranular*. The nonprimary motor areas (the supplementary motor area and the lateral premotor cortex) contain fewer Betz cells than the primary motor areas. The pyramidal cells contribute to two motor pathways important for the production of fine, skilled movements (i.e., movements requiring a precise muscular control), such as those involved in speech and feeding/swallowing and in the movements of the hands. These tracts (often referred to as "pyramidal" tracts in the motor speech literature) are (1) the corticonuclear tracts (historically called *corticobulbar tracts*) that project to the brainstem and cranial motoneurons and (2) the corticospinal tracts that project to the spinal cord and spinal motoneurons. The neurons whose axons form these descending pathways are sometimes called *upper motoneurons*, whereas the cranial or spinal motoneurons they innervate are sometimes called *lower motoneurons*. The majority of the upper motoneurons of the corticonuclear and corticospinal tracts will cross to the contralateral side relative to its origin in the cerebral cortex at the level of the brainstem (Figure 5.5 [p. 215]), but some will remain ipsilateral. There are other motor pathways originating from the cerebral cortex or brainstem that project to cranial and spinal motoneurons, such as the reticulospinal tracts that regulate the control of muscle tone. These are often referred to as "extrapyramidal" tracts in the motor speech literature. Despite the existence of these other descending pathways, the corticonuclear and corticospinal tracts have privileged access to the motoneurons of the brainstem and spinal cord, respectively.

The primary sensory areas, located just caudal to the primary motor area, have an internal organization that is referred to as *granular*. Layering of these areas is also poor but different from the layering of the agranular (motor) areas. Granular areas contain few pyramidal cells and a large number of another type of neuron called *stellar cells*. Primary sensory areas process sensory feedback, including information related to speech, swallowing, and other movements.

Important Sulci

The telencephalon contains the following significant sulci:

- The longitudinal fissure is also referred to as the *sagittal fissure* or *longitudinal cerebral fissure* (Figure 5.4 [p. 214]).
- The lateral sulcus is located on the lateral surface and is also known as the *sylvian fissure* or *fissure of Sylvius* (Figure 5.3 [p. 213]).
- The central sulcus is located on the lateral surface and is also known as the *rolandic fissure* or *fissure of Rolando* (Figure 5.3 [p. 213]).
- The parietooccipital sulcus is located on the medial surface (Figure 5.2 [p. 212]).
- The calcarine sulcus is located on the posteromedial surface (Figures 5.2 [p. 212] and 5.4 [p. 214]).

Cerebral Lobes

The sulci are important landmarks to locate the cerebral lobes. Each hemisphere contains the following four lobes (Figure 5.3 [p. 213]):

1. The frontal lobe is located rostral to the central sulcus and dorsal to the lateral sulcus.
2. The parietal lobe is caudal to the central sulcus. Its caudal limit is an imaginary extension on the lateral surface of the parietooccipital sulcus. The inferior limit is a posterior extension of the sylvian sulcus.
3. The occipital lobe is caudal to the posterior boundary of the parietal lobe, which is an extension of the parietooccipital sulcus.
4. The temporal lobe is inferior to the frontal and parietal lobes and rostral to the occipital lobe.

Internal Surface

The third ventricle is part of the ventricular system, which is a series of ducts that are involved in the production and circulation of cerebrospinal fluid. The corpus callosum (Figure 5.6 [p. 217]) is composed of a collection of axons connecting the two hemispheres. The cingulate gyrus (or cingulum) is located above the corpus callosum (Figure 5.2 [p. 212]). The cingulate gyrus contains a number of anatomically and functionally distinct areas. The cingulate gyrus divides at the level of the anterior commissure into a caudal and a rostral (agranular) region; the latter is involved in movement preparation. Both regions (rostral and caudal) further divide into several functionally distinct areas.

External Surface

The following structures can be identified on the frontal lobe (Figure 5.3 [p. 213]):

- The medial segment of the superior frontal gyrus contains two important motor (agranular) areas that are collectively referred to as the *supplementary motor complex:* (1) the supplementary motor area proper and (2) a more rostral presupplementary motor area. These areas are somatotopically organized and are involved in the production of speech, swallowing, and other movements, especially for the selection, preparation, and initiation in addition to the temporal sequencing of movement components.
- The caudal portion of the precentral gyrus is adjacent to the central sulcus and runs from the lateral sulcus to the mediosuperior surface of the frontal lobe. It contains the agranular primary motor cortex or area. The primary motor cortex is somatotopically organized, with body parts often represented by a distorted body topographical map called a *homunculus.* The face, larynx, and pharynx have a large representation on the inferior portion of the gyrus (Figure 5.5 [p. 215]), reflecting the precision requirements of movements of these structures for speech and feeding/swallowing (and other orofacial movements).
- The anterior portion of the precentral gyrus, near the precentral sulcus, contains the premotor cortex (lateral premotor cortex). The premotor cortex divides into a ventral and a dorsal segment, approximately at the level of the inferior frontal sulcus. Both the ventral and the dorsal premotor area further divide into functionally distinct regions. The premotor cortex is involved in speech (both in production and in perception), swallowing, and other motor behaviors, particularly for the sensorimotor planning of movements, in addition to more cognitive aspects of movement preparation such as response selection.
- The inferior frontal gyrus divides into a ventral orbital area (pars orbitalis), a triangular area (pars triangularis), and a caudal opercular area (pars opercularis). The opercular and triangular regions in the left hemisphere are collectively referred to as the *Broca area* and are involved in the planning and articulation of speech (opercular), in addition to language comprehension, including semantics and syntax (triangular). Brain imaging has revealed swallowing-related activity in the Broca area.

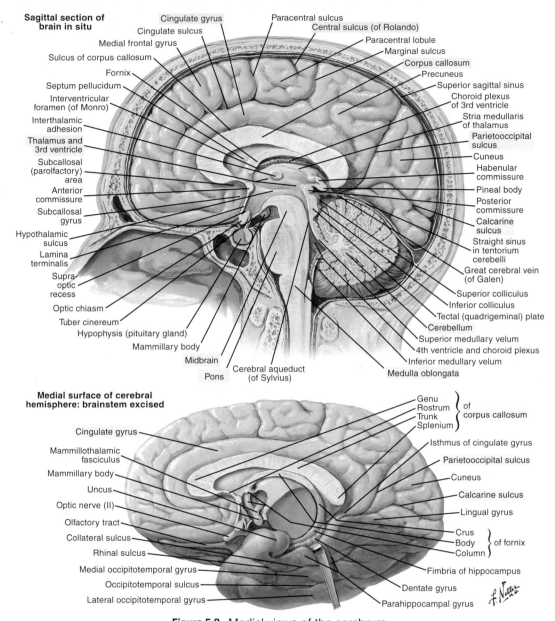

Sagittal section of brain in situ

Cingulate gyrus
Cingulate sulcus
Medial frontal gyrus
Sulcus of corpus callosum
Fornix
Septum pellucidum
Interventricular foramen (of Monro)
Interthalamic adhesion
Thalamus and 3rd ventricle
Subcallosal (parolfactory) area
Anterior commissure
Subcallosal gyrus
Hypothalamic sulcus
Lamina terminalis
Supra-optic recess
Optic chiasm
Tuber cinereum
Hypophysis (pituitary gland)
Mammillary body
Midbrain
Pons
Cerebral aqueduct (of Sylvius)

Paracentral sulcus
Central sulcus (of Rolando)
Paracentral lobule
Marginal sulcus
Corpus callosum
Precuneus
Superior sagittal sinus
Choroid plexus of 3rd ventricle
Stria medullaris of thalamus
Parietooccipital sulcus
Cuneus
Habenular commissure
Pineal body
Posterior commissure
Calcarine sulcus
Straight sinus in tentorium cerebelli
Great cerebral vein (of Galen)
Superior colliculus
Inferior colliculus
Tectal (quadrigeminal) plate
Cerebellum
Superior medullary velum
4th ventricle and choroid plexus
Inferior medullary velum
Medulla oblongata

Medial surface of cerebral hemisphere: brainstem excised

Cingulate gyrus
Mammillothalamic fasciculus
Mammillary body
Uncus
Optic nerve (II)
Olfactory tract
Collateral sulcus
Rhinal sulcus
Medial occipitotemporal gyrus
Occipitotemporal sulcus
Lateral occipitotemporal gyrus

Genu
Rostrum
Trunk
Splenium
} of corpus callosum
Isthmus of cingulate gyrus
Parietooccipital sulcus
Cuneus
Calcarine sulcus
Lingual gyrus
Crus
Body
Column
} of fornix
Fimbria of hippocampus
Dentate gyrus
Parahippocampal gyrus

Figure 5.2. Medial views of the cerebrum.

Note: Labels of certain figures are highlighted in yellow to emphasize the related elements in the corresponding text.

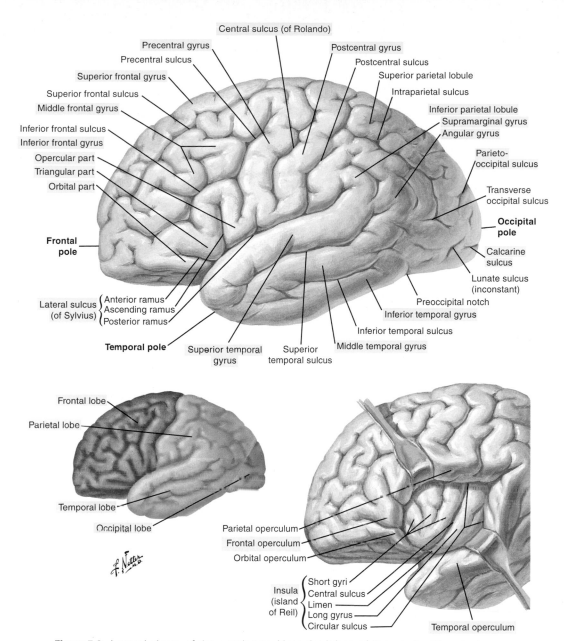

Figure 5.3. Lateral views of the cerebrum. Note the lobes of the cerebral hemispheres.

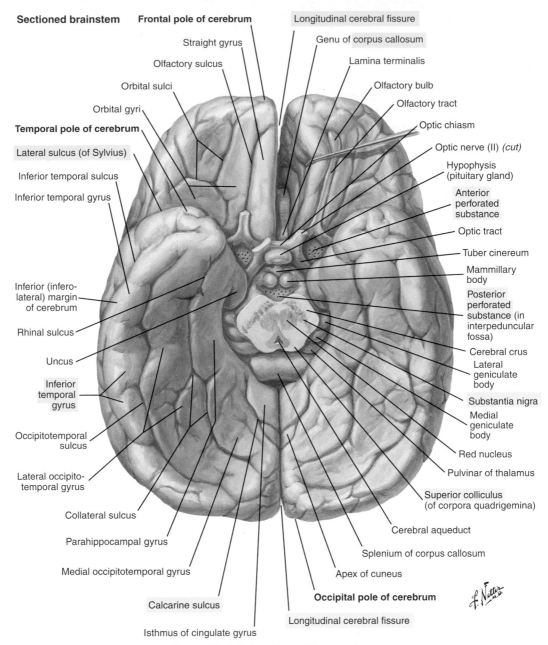

Sectioned brainstem

Frontal pole of cerebrum

Straight gyrus

Olfactory sulcus

Orbital sulci

Orbital gyri

Temporal pole of cerebrum

Lateral sulcus (of Sylvius)

Inferior temporal sulcus

Inferior temporal gyrus

Inferior (infero-
lateral) margin
of cerebrum

Rhinal sulcus

Uncus

Inferior
temporal
gyrus

Occipitotemporal
sulcus

Lateral occipito-
temporal gyrus

Collateral sulcus

Parahippocampal gyrus

Medial occipitotemporal gyrus

Calcarine sulcus

Isthmus of cingulate gyrus

Longitudinal cerebral fissure

Genu of corpus callosum

Lamina terminalis

Olfactory bulb

Olfactory tract

Optic chiasm

Optic nerve (II) (cut)

Hypophysis
(pituitary gland)

Anterior
perforated
substance

Optic tract

Tuber cinereum

Mammillary
body

Posterior
perforated
substance (in
interpeduncular
fossa)

Cerebral crus

Lateral
geniculate
body

Substantia nigra

Medial
geniculate
body

Red nucleus

Pulvinar of thalamus

Superior colliculus
(of corpora quadrigemina)

Cerebral aqueduct

Splenium of corpus callosum

Apex of cuneus

Occipital pole of cerebrum

Longitudinal cerebral fissure

Figure 5.4. Inferior view of the cerebrum.

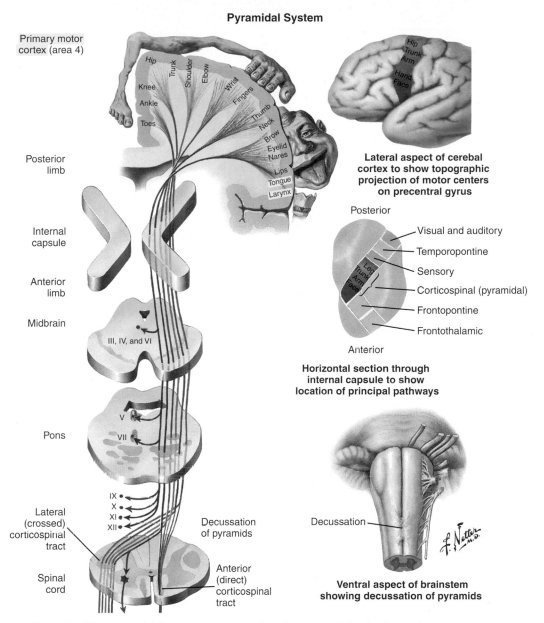

Pyramidal System

Primary motor cortex (area 4)

Hip
Trunk
Shoulder
Elbow
Wrist
Fingers
Thumb
Neck
Brow
Eyelid
Nares
Lips
Tongue
Larynx
Knee
Ankle
Toes

Posterior limb

Internal capsule

Anterior limb

Midbrain

III, IV, and VI

Pons

V

VII

IX
X
XI
XII

Lateral (crossed) corticospinal tract

Spinal cord

Decussation of pyramids

Anterior (direct) corticospinal tract

Hip
Trunk
Arm
Hand
Face

Lateral aspect of cerebral cortex to show topographic projection of motor centers on precentral gyrus

Posterior

Visual and auditory

Temporopontine

Sensory

Corticospinal (pyramidal)

Frontopontine

Frontothalamic

Leg
Trunk
Arm
Face

Anterior

Horizontal section through internal capsule to show location of principal pathways

Decussation

Ventral aspect of brainstem showing decussation of pyramids

Figure 5.5. The pyramidal system, representing the parts of the body on the motor cortex.

The following structures can be identified on the parietal lobe (see Figure 5.3 [p. 213]):

- The postcentral gyrus (located posterior or caudal to the central sulcus) is important for the processing of sensory information; thus it is called the *primary sensory (somatosensory) cortex* or *area*. Similar to the primary motor cortex, body parts are topographically represented in the primary sensory cortex.
- The supramarginal gyrus is located around the caudal border of the lateral fissure.
- The angular gyrus is located around the caudal border of the superior temporal sulcus.

These two areas, the supramarginal gyrus and the angular gyrus, receive auditory, visual, and somatosensory information. The supramarginal gyrus participates in phonological processing, and the angular gyrus is involved in semantic processing.

The following structures can be identified on the temporal lobe (see Figure 5.3 [p. 213]):

- The superior, middle, and inferior temporal gyri are located here. The *temporal operculum* is formed by the superior temporal and transverse temporal gyri. Operculum means "lid," and in this case it covers the insula.
- The Heschl's gyrus (not shown in Figure 5.3) is located deep within the lateral sulcus on the temporal operculum. The Heschl's gyrus contains the primary auditory cortex or area.
- The planum temporale is located on the temporal operculum, posterior to the Heschl's gyrus.
- The Wernicke's area is on the posterior half of the superior temporal gyrus of the left hemisphere and includes the planum temporale. This area is important for language, particularly for language comprehension.
- The gustatory cortex is located on the frontal operculum and anterior insular cortex. This area is involved in the integration of olfactory and gustatory sensory inputs for food ingestion.
- The insular cortex (insula) is located deep within the lateral sulcus and is composed of the anterior and posterior insular cortices. Brain imaging and electrical stimulation data have revealed activation of the insula for speech and swallowing movements.

Internal Structures of the Cerebral Hemispheres

Underneath the cortex, the following structures can be found:

- White matter tracts connecting different parts of the cortex or traveling to or from the brainstem and spinal cord
- The hippocampal formation, the amygdala, and the basal ganglia

Basal Ganglia

The basal ganglia contain the following (Figure 5.6):

Anatomical structures
- Caudate nucleus
- Putamen
- Globus pallidus (external and internal segments)

Functional components
- Substantia nigra
- Subthalamic nucleus

The basal ganglia, which are located deep in the telencephalon, are also known as the *basal nuclei*. They participate in the control of body posture and muscle tone and in planning and initiating movements. The putamen and globus pallidus are collectively referred to as the *lentiform* or *lenticular nucleus*. The caudate nucleus and the putamen together form the *striate body* or the corpus striatum. The substantia nigra (midbrain) and subthalamic nuclei (diencephalon), although not anatomically located in the telencephalon, are often considered to be functional components of the basal ganglia.

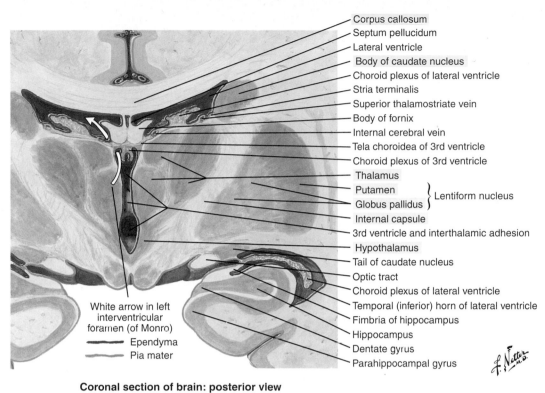

Corpus callosum
Septum pellucidum
Lateral ventricle
Body of caudate nucleus
Choroid plexus of lateral ventricle
Stria terminalis
Superior thalamostriate vein
Body of fornix
Internal cerebral vein
Tela choroidea of 3rd ventricle
Choroid plexus of 3rd ventricle
Thalamus
Putamen
Globus pallidus } Lentiform nucleus
Internal capsule
3rd ventricle and interthalamic adhesion
Hypothalamus
Tail of caudate nucleus
Optic tract
Choroid plexus of lateral ventricle
Temporal (inferior) horn of lateral ventricle
Fimbria of hippocampus
Hippocampus
Dentate gyrus
Parahippocampal gyrus

White arrow in left
interventricular
foramen (of Monro)
Ependyma
Pia mater

Coronal section of brain: posterior view

Figure 5.6. A coronal section of the basal ganglia, thalamus, and associated structures.

■ DIENCEPHALON (THALAMUS, HYPOTHALAMUS, EPITHALAMUS, AND SUBTHALAMUS) (see Figure 5.6 [p. 217])

Characteristic Features

The diencephalon is located deep in and almost entirely encircled by the cerebral hemispheres. It contains the following structures: (1) thalamus, (2) hypothalamus, (3) epithalamus, and (4) subthalamus.

Importance for Speech and Swallowing

The thalamus contains multiple nuclei that are part of motor, sensory, and associative pathways. The thalamus receives all sensory feedback, with the exception of olfactory feedback, and relays this information to the cortex. Because of this, it is often considered only as sensory relay nuclei. However, the thalamus has reciprocal connections with the cortex, receiving not only sensory feedback but also motor signals, indicating an additional role in movement production.

The ventrolateral nucleus and the ventroanterior nucleus connect the basal ganglia and cerebellum to their respective motor and premotor cortices and are consequently involved in motor planning and initiation of movement.

■ MESENCEPHALON (MIDBRAIN) (see Figures 5.2 [p. 212] and 5.4 [p. 214])

Characteristic Features

The mesencephalon is the smallest portion of the brainstem and is located just above the pons. It contains a number of nuclei, including the substantia nigra (part of the basal ganglia) and the inferior and superior colliculi, which are collectively referred to as the *corpora quadrigemina*. Inferior colliculi are important central auditory pathway nuclei, and superior colliculi are important central visual pathway nuclei.

Fibers from the corticospinal, corticonuclear, and corticopontine tracts pass through the mesencephalon. The base of the mesencephalon includes the superior cerebellar peduncles.

Importance for Speech and Swallowing

The substantia nigra has an important role in regulating motor activity, particularly in initiating and terminating movements. The mesencephalon houses the nuclei of several cranial nerves (see the section "Cranial Nerves," pp. 239–257). The inferior colliculi are important auditory relay and processing nuclei.

■ METENCEPHALON (PONS AND CEREBELLUM) (Figure 5.7; see also Figure 5.2 [p. 212])

Characteristic Features

The metencephalon is composed of the pons and cerebellum (discussed in more detail later). The pons contains vertical and horizontal fibers. The horizontal fibers are located on the anterior surface of the pons and form the cerebellar peduncles, which connect the brainstem to the cerebellum. The vertical (longitudinal) fibers of the metencephalon are continuous with the myelencephalon longitudinal fibers and carry sensory and motor information.

Importance for Speech and Swallowing

The pons contains the motor nuclei of two cranial nerves important for speech and swallowing: the trigeminal nerve (V) and the facial nerve (VII).

■ MYELENCEPHALON (MEDULLA OBLONGATA) (Figure 5.7; see also Figure 5.2 [p. 212])

Characteristic Features

The medulla is the most caudal portion of the brainstem. It is located between the pons and the spinal cord, ventral to the cerebellum. The medulla resembles an enlargement of the spinal cord.

Importance for Speech and Swallowing

The medulla contains the nucleus ambiguus, which contains the motor nuclei of cranial nerves important for speech and swallowing: the glossopharyngeal (IX) and the vagus (X). Although the nucleus ambiguus receives inputs from both cerebral hemispheres, the majority comes from the contralateral hemisphere.

Brainstem Central Pattern Generators

The pons and medulla contain important pattern-generating nuclei, sometimes called brainstem *central pattern generators* (CPGs). This term is used because these collections of neurons contain the neural circuitry needed to generate some fundamental rhythmic and repetitive movements such as swallowing, mastication, respiration, and locomotion. The pattern generators for these movements may share multifunctional neurons that are biased to produce one or the other behavior (or coordinate the two, in the case of breathing and swallowing, for example). Although basic patterns can be generated by brainstem nuclei alone, adapting movements to changing external or internal environmental conditions (for example, different types of food boluses) requires sensory feedback and inputs from higher levels of the nervous system (e.g., cortical inputs). Thus the CPGs are only a portion of the complex neural machinery controlling these complex behaviors. It has also been suggested that speech production uses, or "fractionates," some of the brainstem circuitry for breathing, mastication, and swallowing for the production of speech.

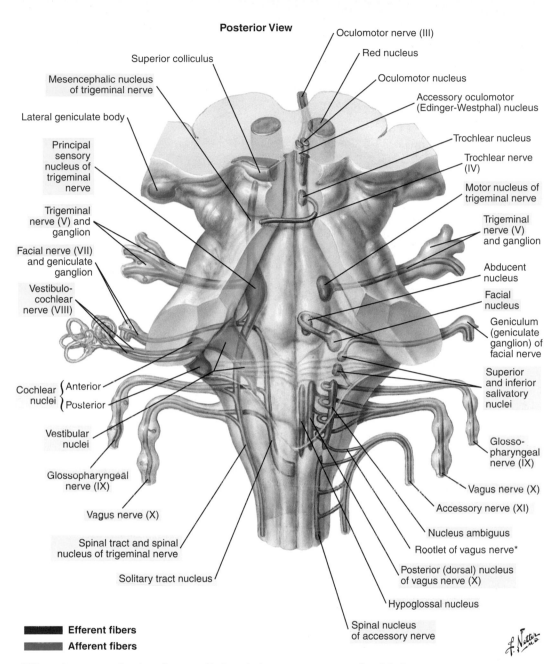

Posterior View

Oculomotor nerve (III)

Superior colliculus

Red nucleus

Mesencephalic nucleus
of trigeminal nerve

Oculomotor nucleus

Accessory oculomotor
(Edinger-Westphal) nucleus

Lateral geniculate body

Trochlear nucleus

Principal
sensory
nucleus of
trigeminal
nerve

Trochlear nerve
(IV)

Motor nucleus of
trigeminal nerve

Trigeminal
nerve (V) and
ganglion

Trigeminal
nerve (V)
and ganglion

Facial nerve (VII)
and geniculate
ganglion

Abducent
nucleus

Vestibulo-
cochlear
nerve (VIII)

Facial
nucleus

Geniculum
(geniculate
ganglion) of
facial nerve

Cochlear { Anterior
nuclei { Posterior

Superior
and inferior
salivatory
nuclei

Vestibular
nuclei

Glosso-
pharyngeal
nerve (IX)

Glossopharyngeal
nerve (IX)

Vagus nerve (X)

Vagus nerve (X)

Accessory nerve (XI)

Spinal tract and spinal
nucleus of trigeminal nerve

Nucleus ambiguus

Rootlet of vagus nerve*

Solitary tract nucleus

Posterior (dorsal) nucleus
of vagus nerve (X)

Hypoglossal nucleus

Spinal nucleus
of accessory nerve

■■■■ **Efferent fibers**
■■■■ **Afferent fibers**

*This rootlet may travel a short distance with the spinal accessory to eventually rejoin the vagus.

Figure 5.7. The location of the cranial nerve nuclei and their afferent *(blue)* and efferent *(red)* fiber tracts in the brainstem.

■ SPINAL CORD (Figure 5.8)

Characteristic Features

The spinal cord is the elongated, nearly cylindrical part of the central nervous system contained within the vertebral column. The superior boundary of the spinal cord is the base of the medulla, and its inferior boundary is the first or second lumbar vertebra. The spinal cord is protected by the vertebral column and the spinal meninges. It is divided into 31 segments, and each segment gives rise to a ventral root (efferent) and a dorsal root (afferent), which fuse to form a spinal nerve (see the section "Spinal Nerves," p. 258).

Internal Structures

In a cross-section of the spinal cord, the following structures can be seen:
- The butterfly-shaped gray matter is located deep into the cord.
- The white matter surrounds the gray matter and contains ascending and descending pathways. The white matter pathways carry information from the brain to the periphery (motor) and from the periphery to the brain (sensory).

Spinal Cord Cross-Sections: Fiber Tracts

Sections through spinal cord at various levels

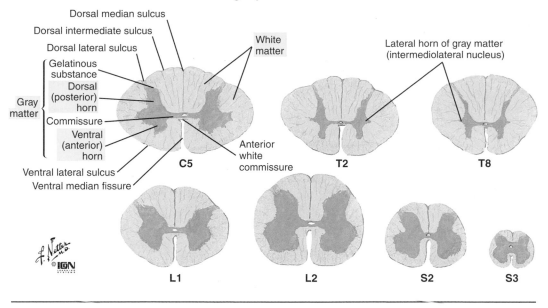

Dorsal median sulcus
Dorsal intermediate sulcus
Dorsal lateral sulcus
Gelatinous substance
Dorsal (posterior) horn
Gray matter
Commissure
Ventral (anterior) horn
Ventral lateral sulcus
Ventral median fissure
White matter
Anterior white commissure
C5

Lateral horn of gray matter (intermediolateral nucleus)
T2
T8

L1
L2
S2
S3

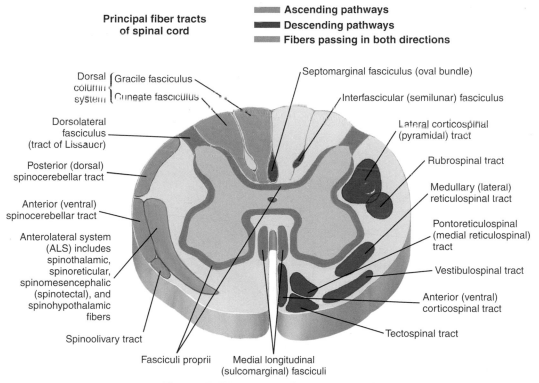

Principal fiber tracts of spinal cord

- ▬ **Ascending pathways**
- ▬ **Descending pathways**
- ▬ **Fibers passing in both directions**

Dorsal column system
 {Gracile fasciculus
  Cuneate fasciculus

Dorsolateral fasciculus (tract of Lissauer)

Posterior (dorsal) spinocerebellar tract

Anterior (ventral) spinocerebellar tract

Anterolateral system (ALS) includes spinothalamic, spinoreticular, spinomesencephalic (spinotectal), and spinohypothalamic fibers

Spinoolivary tract

Fasciculi proprii

Medial longitudinal (sulcomarginal) fasciculi

Septomarginal fasciculus (oval bundle)

Interfascicular (semilunar) fasciculus

Lateral corticospinal (pyramidal) tract

Rubrospinal tract

Medullary (lateral) reticulospinal tract

Pontoreticulospinal (medial reticulospinal) tract

Vestibulospinal tract

Anterior (ventral) corticospinal tract

Tectospinal tract

Figure 5.8. Fiber tracts of the spinal cord.

■ CEREBELLUM (Figures 5.9 and 5.10 [p. 226])

Characteristic Features

The cerebellum ("small brain") is a complex anatomical structure located posterior to the pons and medulla and inferior to the occipital lobe, which partially overlaps it. It is connected to the brainstem and to the rest of the brain through the inferior, middle, and superior peduncles that contain afferent and efferent fibers. We are still discovering the potential roles of the cerebellum in speech and swallowing, but like other complex movements, it is likely that it participates in movement planning and regulation in addition to motor learning and memory.

The cerebellum is composed of an external layer (the cerebellar cortex) of gray matter, an internal core of white matter, and several deep nuclei, including (from lateral to medial) the dentate, interposed (composed of the globose and emboliform nuclei), and fastigial nuclei. These act as relay nuclei for efferent and afferent cerebellar pathways. A sagittal section through the cerebellum (Figure 5.10 [p. 226]) reveals its treelike structure originally referred to as the *arbor vitae,* or "tree of life." Also apparent in transverse section is the complex surface structure of the cerebellar cortex that, unlike the gyri of the cerebral cortex, resembles "leaves" of a tree and are thus named *folia.*

The cerebellum has a midline structure called the *vermis* that connects the two cerebellar hemispheres. Each hemisphere is divided into three lobes: anterior, posterior, and flocculonodular.

The cerebellum can be further divided into three functional and phylogenetic (from the evolutionary oldest to the most recent) regions (Figure 5.11 [p. 227]): the vestibulocerebellum (or archicerebellum), which corresponds to the flocculonodular lobes; the spinocerebellum (or paleocerebellum), which includes the vermis and paravermis regions; and the cerebrocerebellum (or neocerebellum), which includes the lateral portions of both the anterior and posterior lobes.

The vestibulocerebellum, which receives inputs from and projects to the vestibular nuclei, is implicated in the regulation of posture and balance. Efferent pathways help coordinate eye, head, and body movements in response to information from the semicircular canals and otolithic organs in the inner ear.

The spinocerebellum receives proprioceptive afferent inputs from the spinal cord and trigeminal system. Projections from cerebellar deep nuclei (interposed and fastigial) regulate muscle tone and posture via subcortical upper motor neuron pathways. Both motor outputs and sensory inputs are somatotopically organized in the spinocerebellum.

The cerebrocerebellum (or pontocerebellum) is involved in the planning, initiation, and regulation of skilled movements, including speech. The cerebrocerebellum receives input indirectly from the cerebral cortex and projects from the dentate nucleus to the premotor and association cortices of the frontal lobes via the thalamus.

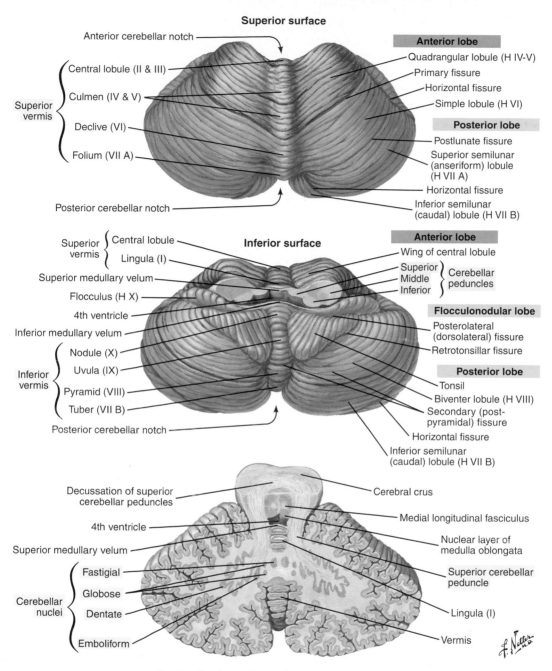

Superior surface

Anterior cerebellar notch

Anterior lobe

Central lobule (II & III)

Culmen (IV & V)

Superior vermis

Declive (VI)

Folium (VII A)

Quadrangular lobule (H IV-V)

Primary fissure

Horizontal fissure

Simple lobule (H VI)

Posterior lobe

Postlunate fissure

Superior semilunar (anseriform) lobule (H VII A)

Horizontal fissure

Posterior cerebellar notch

Inferior semilunar (caudal) lobule (H VII B)

Inferior surface

Superior vermis { Central lobule

Lingula (I)

Superior medullary velum

Flocculus (H X)

4th ventricle

Inferior medullary velum

Inferior vermis { Nodule (X)

Uvula (IX)

Pyramid (VIII)

Tuber (VII B)

Posterior cerebellar notch

Anterior lobe

Wing of central lobule

Superior
Middle
Inferior } Cerebellar peduncles

Flocculonodular lobe

Posterolateral (dorsolateral) fissure

Retrotonsillar fissure

Posterior lobe

Tonsil

Biventer lobule (H VIII)

Secondary (post-pyramidal) fissure

Horizontal fissure

Inferior semilunar (caudal) lobule (H VII B)

Decussation of superior cerebellar peduncles

4th ventricle

Superior medullary velum

Cerebellar nuclei { Fastigial

Globose

Dentate

Emboliform

Cerebral crus

Medial longitudinal fasciculus

Nuclear layer of medulla oblongata

Superior cerebellar peduncle

Lingula (I)

Vermis

Section in plane of superior cerebellar peduncle

Figure 5.9. The cerebellum.

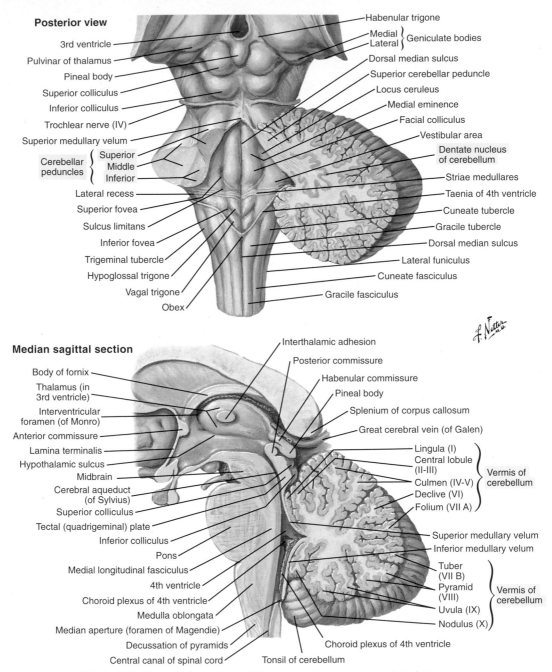

Posterior view

Habenular trigone

3rd ventricle

Medial } Geniculate bodies
Lateral

Pulvinar of thalamus

Dorsal median sulcus

Pineal body

Superior cerebellar peduncle

Superior colliculus

Locus ceruleus

Inferior colliculus

Medial eminence

Trochlear nerve (IV)

Facial colliculus

Superior medullary velum

Vestibular area

Cerebellar
peduncles { Superior
Middle
Inferior

Dentate nucleus
of cerebellum

Striae medullares

Lateral recess

Taenia of 4th ventricle

Superior fovea

Cuneate tubercle

Sulcus limitans

Gracile tubercle

Inferior fovea

Dorsal median sulcus

Trigeminal tubercle

Lateral funiculus

Hypoglossal trigone

Cuneate fasciculus

Vagal trigone

Gracile fasciculus

Obex

f. Netter

Median sagittal section

Interthalamic adhesion

Posterior commissure

Body of fornix

Habenular commissure

Thalamus (in
3rd ventricle)

Pineal body

Interventricular
foramen (of Monro)

Splenium of corpus callosum

Anterior commissure

Great cerebral vein (of Galen)

Lamina terminalis

Lingula (I)
Central lobule
(II-III) } Vermis of
cerebellum

Hypothalamic sulcus

Midbrain

Culmen (IV-V)

Cerebral aqueduct
(of Sylvius)

Declive (VI)

Superior colliculus

Folium (VII A)

Tectal (quadrigeminal) plate

Superior medullary velum

Inferior colliculus

Inferior medullary velum

Pons

Tuber
(VII B)

Medial longitudinal fasciculus

Pyramid
(VIII) } Vermis of
cerebellum

4th ventricle

Choroid plexus of 4th ventricle

Uvula (IX)

Medulla oblongata

Nodulus (X)

Median aperture (foramen of Magendie)

Choroid plexus of 4th ventricle

Decussation of pyramids

Central canal of spinal cord

Tonsil of cerebellum

Figure 5.10. A sagittal section of the cerebellum and associated structures.

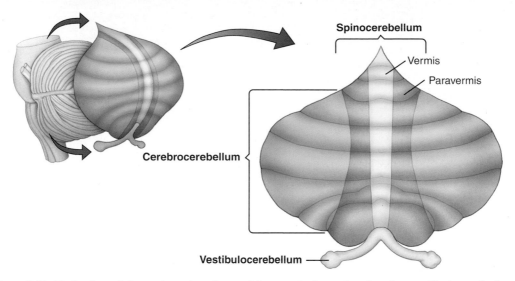

Figure 5.11. Flattening of the external surface of the cerebellum showing the vestibulocerebellum, spinocerebellum, and cerebrocerebellum (or pontocerebellum) regions. (Redrawn from Purves D, Augustine GJ, Fitzpatrick D, et al: *Neuroscience*, ed 5, Sunderland, MA, 2012, Sinauer Associates, Inc., Publishers.)

■ MENINGES (Figure 5.12)

The following three layers of protective coatings surround the brain (and spinal cord):
1. Dura mater
2. Arachnoid mater
3. Pia mater

Dura Mater

The dura mater has a tough outer fibrous layer, which is actually two layers (inner meningeal and outer periosteal) that are contiguous except where they separate to accommodate the dural venous sinuses (e.g., superior sagittal sinus).

Arachnoid Mater

The arachnoid mater is the medial layer and is much thinner than the dura mater. It follows the convolutions of the brain, but not as closely as the pia mater. The subarachnoid space, located between the arachnoid and the pia mater, contains cerebrospinal fluid.

Pia Mater

The pia mater is the deepest and extremely thin layer that closely follows the brain's surface and tightly covers fissures and sulci. The arachnoid and pia mater together are referred to as the *leptomeninges*.

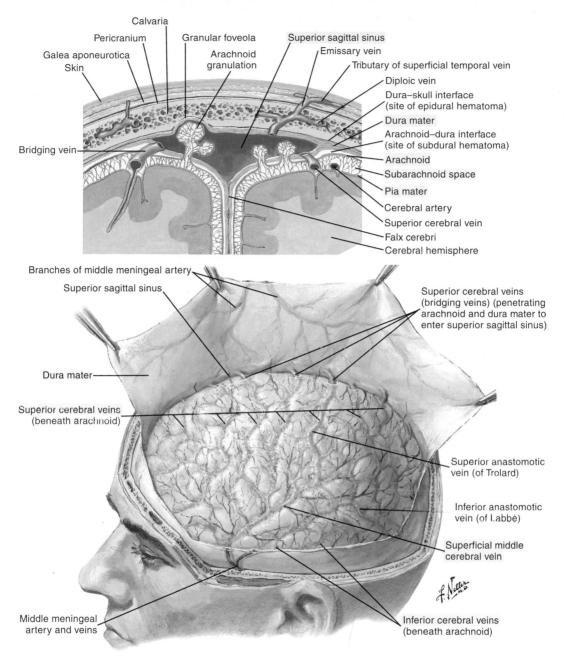

Figure 5.12. The meninges and superficial cerebral veins.

■ CEREBROSPINAL FLUID (Figures 5.13 and 5.14 [p. 232])

The principal source of cerebrospinal fluid is the choroid plexuses in the lateral ventricles, with contributions from other ventricular and extraventricular sites. Cerebrospinal fluid flows from the third and fourth ventricles into the subarachnoid space. It is reabsorbed into the dural venous sinuses and other sites and supports the weight of the brain and provides shock absorption against brain trauma. Cerebrospinal fluid transports nutrients and eliminates waste products.

Left lateral phantom view

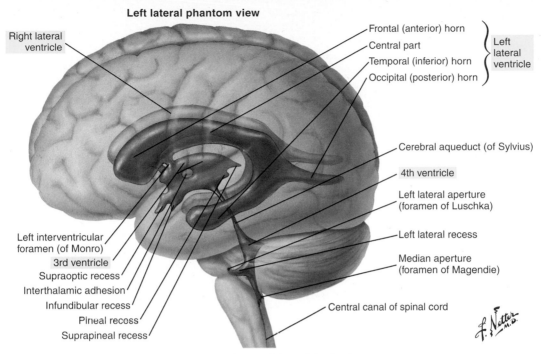

Right lateral ventricle

Frontal (anterior) horn

Central part

Temporal (inferior) horn

Occipital (posterior) horn

Left lateral ventricle

Cerebral aqueduct (of Sylvius)

4th ventricle

Left lateral aperture (foramen of Luschka)

Left lateral recess

Median aperture (foramen of Magendie)

Left interventricular foramen (of Monro)

3rd ventricle

Supraoptic recess

Interthalamic adhesion

Infundibular recess

Pineal recess

Suprapineal recess

Central canal of spinal cord

Figure 5.13. Ventricles of the brain.

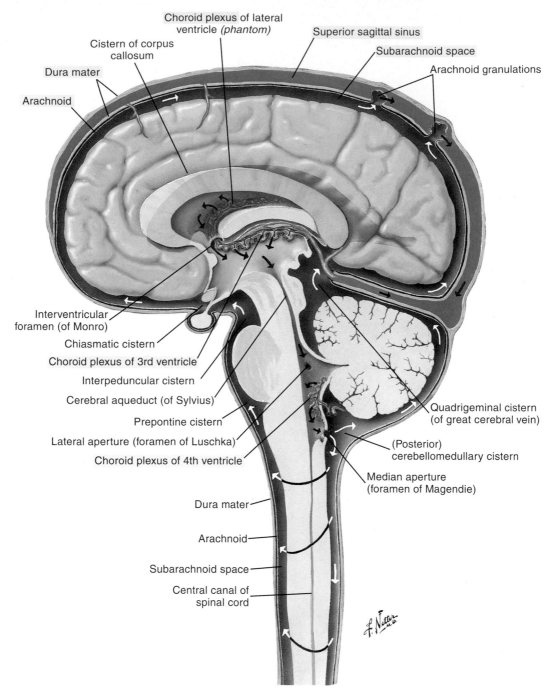

Choroid plexus of lateral
ventricle *(phantom)*

Superior sagittal sinus

Subarachnoid space

Arachnoid granulations

Cistern of corpus
callosum

Dura mater

Arachnoid

Interventricular
foramen (of Monro)

Chiasmatic cistern

Choroid plexus of 3rd ventricle

Interpeduncular cistern

Cerebral aqueduct (of Sylvius)

Prepontine cistern

Lateral aperture (foramen of Luschka)

Choroid plexus of 4th ventricle

Quadrigeminal cistern
(of great cerebral vein)

(Posterior)
cerebellomedullary cistern

Median aperture
(foramen of Magendie)

Dura mater

Arachnoid

Subarachnoid space

Central canal of
spinal cord

Figure 5.14. The circulation of cerebrospinal fluid.

■ CEREBRAL CIRCULATION (Figures 5.15 [p. 234], 5.16 [p. 235], and 5.17 [p. 236]; see also Figure 5.12 [p. 229])

Vascular Supply

Brain tissues have a high metabolic rate, and appropriate blood flow is crucial. The brain consumes approximately 25% of the oxygen supply of the body.

Vascular supply of the brain is provided by the internal carotid arteries (branches of the common carotid arteries) and the vertebral arteries (branches of the subclavian arteries). These arteries subdivide to ensure blood supply to the entire brain. The internal carotid arteries give rise to the anterior cerebral arteries and the middle cerebral arteries. The vertebral arteries merge at the level of the pons to become the basilar artery and then bifurcate to become the posterior cerebral arteries. The vertebral arteries and the basilar artery are responsible for the blood supply of the brainstem and cerebellum.

- The anterior cerebral arteries subdivide into cortical and central branches. The cortical branches supply the superior and medial portions of the cortex (including the superior frontal gyri, medial frontal gyri, cingulate gyri, precuneus, and corpus callosum). The central branches enter the anterior perforated substance (see Figure 5.4 [p. 214]) and contribute to the blood supply of internal structures, including the inferior and anterior portions of the basal ganglia (part of the putamen and of the head of the caudate nucleus) in addition to the adjacent regions of the internal capsules.
- The middle cerebral arteries divide into cortical and central branches. Cortical branches supply most of the lateral surfaces of the cerebral hemispheres (including the middle and inferior frontal gyri, the superior and middle temporal gyri, the supramarginal and angular gyri, the inferior portion of the precentral and postcentral gyri, and the insula). Central branches enter the anterior perforated substance to contribute to the blood supply of the internal structures, including the superior portions of the basal ganglia (portions of the lentiform nucleus and upper parts of the head and body of the caudate nucleus) and the superior portions of the internal capsules (Figure 5.16 [p. 235] – bottom figure).
- Cortical branches of the posterior cerebral arteries supply the occipital lobe, most of the inferior temporal gyri, and part of the inferior surface of the cerebral hemispheres (including the parahippocampal, medial occipitotemporal, and lateral occipitotemporal gyri). Central branches of the posterior cerebral arteries enter the posterior perforated substance (see Figure 5.4 [p. 214]) to supply blood to the thalamus and the midbrain.

Circle of Willis

The *circle of Willis* (Figure 5.18 [p. 237]) is a key distribution network for blood to the brain. It is formed by the basilar artery, internal carotid arteries, middle cerebral arteries, anterior cerebral arteries, anterior communicating arteries that join the right and left anterior cerebral arteries, and posterior cerebral arteries that join the internal carotids by the posterior communicating arteries. Thus, through the communicating arteries, this vasculature forms a circle of blood flow to the brain and allows for collateral blood flow in the event of interruptions to cerebral vasculature as the result of disease or damage (e.g., stroke).

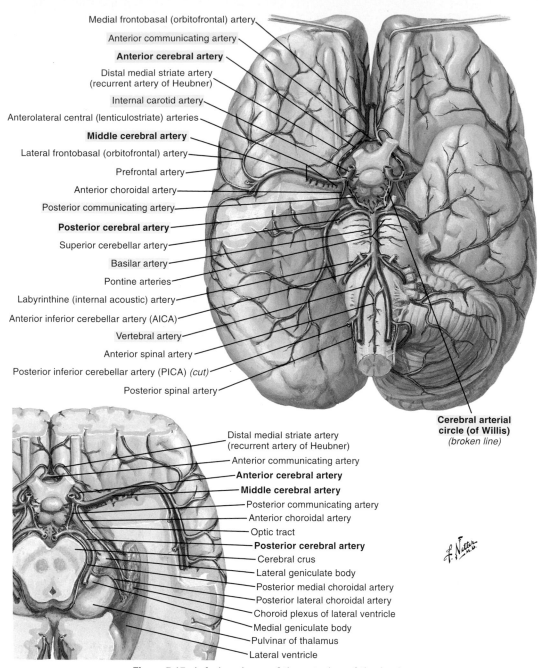

Medial frontobasal (orbitofrontal) artery

Anterior communicating artery

Anterior cerebral artery

Distal medial striate artery
(recurrent artery of Heubner)

Internal carotid artery

Anterolateral central (lenticulostriate) arteries

Middle cerebral artery

Lateral frontobasal (orbitofrontal) artery

Prefrontal artery

Anterior choroidal artery

Posterior communicating artery

Posterior cerebral artery

Superior cerebellar artery

Basilar artery

Pontine arteries

Labyrinthine (internal acoustic) artery

Anterior inferior cerebellar artery (AICA)

Vertebral artery

Anterior spinal artery

Posterior inferior cerebellar artery (PICA) *(cut)*

Posterior spinal artery

**Cerebral arterial
circle (of Willis)**
(broken line)

Distal medial striate artery
(recurrent artery of Heubner)

Anterior communicating artery

Anterior cerebral artery

Middle cerebral artery

Posterior communicating artery

Anterior choroidal artery

Optic tract

Posterior cerebral artery

Cerebral crus

Lateral geniculate body

Posterior medial choroidal artery

Posterior lateral choroidal artery

Choroid plexus of lateral ventricle

Medial geniculate body

Pulvinar of thalamus

Lateral ventricle

Figure 5.15. Inferior views of the arteries of the brain.

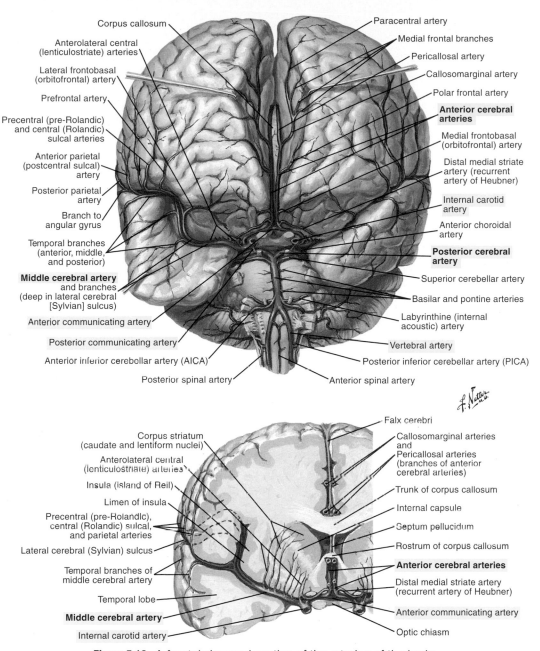

Corpus callosum

Anterolateral central (lenticulostriate) arteries

Lateral frontobasal (orbitofrontal) artery

Prefrontal artery

Precentral (pre-Rolandic) and central (Rolandic) sulcal arteries

Anterior parietal (postcentral sulcal) artery

Posterior parietal artery

Branch to angular gyrus

Temporal branches (anterior, middle, and posterior)

Middle cerebral artery and branches (deep in lateral cerebral [Sylvian] sulcus)

Anterior communicating artery

Posterior communicating artery

Anterior inferior cerebellar artery (AICA)

Posterior spinal artery

Paracentral artery

Medial frontal branches

Pericallosal artery

Callosomarginal artery

Polar frontal artery

Anterior cerebral arteries

Medial frontobasal (orbitofrontal) artery

Distal medial striate artery (recurrent artery of Heubner)

Internal carotid artery

Anterior choroidal artery

Posterior cerebral artery

Superior cerebellar artery

Basilar and pontine arteries

Labyrinthine (internal acoustic) artery

Vertebral artery

Posterior inferior cerebellar artery (PICA)

Anterior spinal artery

Corpus striatum (caudate and lentiform nuclei)

Anterolateral central (lenticulostriate) arteries

Insula (island of Reil)

Limen of insula

Precentral (pre-Rolandic), central (Rolandic) sulcal, and parietal arteries

Lateral cerebral (Sylvian) sulcus

Temporal branches of middle cerebral artery

Temporal lobe

Middle cerebral artery

Internal carotid artery

Falx cerebri

Callosomarginal arteries and Pericallosal arteries (branches of anterior cerebral arteries)

Trunk of corpus callosum

Internal capsule

Septum pellucidum

Rostrum of corpus callosum

Anterior cerebral arteries

Distal medial striate artery (recurrent artery of Heubner)

Anterior communicating artery

Optic chiasm

Figure 5.16. A frontal view and section of the arteries of the brain.

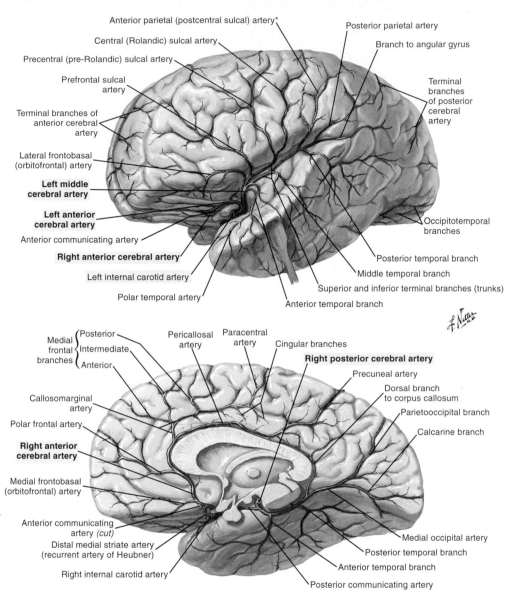

Anterior parietal (postcentral sulcal) artery*

Central (Rolandic) sulcal artery

Precentral (pre-Rolandic) sulcal artery

Prefrontal sulcal artery

Terminal branches of anterior cerebral artery

Lateral frontobasal (orbitofrontal) artery

Left middle cerebral artery

Left anterior cerebral artery

Anterior communicating artery

Right anterior cerebral artery

Left internal carotid artery

Polar temporal artery

Posterior parietal artery

Branch to angular gyrus

Terminal branches of posterior cerebral artery

Occipitotemporal branches

Posterior temporal branch

Middle temporal branch

Superior and inferior terminal branches (trunks)

Anterior temporal branch

Medial frontal branches { Posterior, Intermediate, Anterior

Pericallosal artery

Paracentral artery

Cingular branches

Right posterior cerebral artery

Precuneal artery

Dorsal branch to corpus callosum

Parietooccipital branch

Calcarine branch

Callosomarginal artery

Polar frontal artery

Right anterior cerebral artery

Medial frontobasal (orbitofrontal) artery

Anterior communicating artery (cut)

Distal medial striate artery (recurrent artery of Heubner)

Right internal carotid artery

Medial occipital artery

Posterior temporal branch

Anterior temporal branch

Posterior communicating artery

*Note: Anterior parietal (postcentral sulcal) artery also occurs as separate anterior parietal and postcentral sulcal arteries.

Figure 5.17. Lateral and medial views of the arteries of the brain.

Vessels dissected out: inferior view

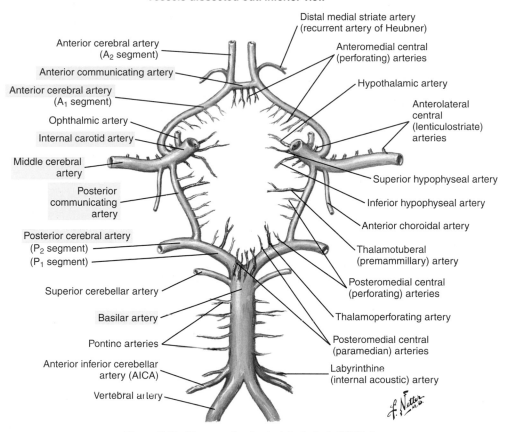

Anterior cerebral artery
(A₂ segment)

Anterior communicating artery

Anterior cerebral artery
(A₁ segment)

Ophthalmic artery

Internal carotid artery

Middle cerebral
artery

Posterior
communicating
artery

Posterior cerebral artery
(P₂ segment)
(P₁ segment)

Superior cerebellar artery

Basilar artery

Pontine arteries

Anterior inferior cerebellar
artery (AICA)

Vertebral artery

Distal medial striate artery
(recurrent artery of Heubner)

Anteromedial central
(perforating) arteries

Hypothalamic artery

Anterolateral
central
(lenticulostriate)
arteries

Superior hypophyseal artery

Inferior hypophyseal artery

Anterior choroidal artery

Thalamotuberal
(premammillary) artery

Posteromedial central
(perforating) arteries

Thalamoperforating artery

Posteromedial central
(paramedian) arteries

Labyrinthine
(internal acoustic) artery

Figure 5.18. The cerebral arterial circle (of Willis).

Venous Drainage

A system of superficial and deep veins ensures venous drainage of the brain. Superior and inferior cerebral veins, in addition to the superficial middle cerebral veins, participate in the venous drainage of the cerebral cortex. The internal cerebral veins, the basal veins, and the great cerebral vein are involved in the drainage of the midbrain and deep structures of the cerebral hemispheres (for example, the insula, thalamus, and basal ganglia). Superior and inferior cerebellar veins participate in the drainage of the cerebellum.

The veins cross the arachnoid and the inner meningeal layer of the dura mater and converge to the dural venous sinuses, the spaces between the two layers of the dura mater (see Figures 5.12 [p. 229] and 5.14 [p. 232]). Most of the venous blood is drained from the venous sinuses to the internal jugular veins.

■ NERVES

The peripheral nervous system includes the cranial nerves and the spinal nerves. A nerve is composed of nerve fibers surrounded by connective tissue. Depending on its function, a nerve contains motor fibers, sensory fibers, or a combination of both.

Types of Nerve Fibers

Cranial and spinal nerves can carry up to six functionally distinct types of fibers: three types of sensory fibers and three types of motor fibers. The terms *afferent* for sensory and *efferent* for motor are often used.

Sensory Fibers
- General sensory fibers carry touch, pain, temperature, and proprioception.
- Special sensory fibers carry hearing, balance, vision, taste, and smell; they are sometimes divided into special somatic (hearing, vision, and balance) and special visceral (smell and taste). They are found only in some cranial nerves.
- Visceral sensory fibers carry sensory information (except pain) from the viscera.

Motor Fibers
- Somatic motor fibers innervate somatic skeletal muscles.
- Branchial motor fibers innervate skeletal muscles that develop from the branchial arches (branchiomeric). They are found only in some cranial nerves.
- Visceral motor (parasympathetic efferent) fibers innervate smooth muscles and glands.

Cerebral Cortex Innervation of Cranial and Spinal Nerves

The neural control of speech and swallowing is potentially different from the neural control of the limbs. Oropharyngeal movements, such as speech and swallowing, require the precise, bilateral activation of median paired muscles (e.g., the intrinsic tongue muscles). Because of this, cranial nerves potentially receive more bilateral innervation from cortical pathways than spinal nerves. For example, portions of the facial and hypoglossal cranial nerves receive greater bilateral (coming from the two cerebral hemispheres) than contralateral (coming from the opposite hemisphere) innervation. In contrast, spinal nerves controlling limb movements receive predominantly contralateral innervation.

■ CRANIAL NERVES (Figures 5.19 [p. 240], 5.20 [p. 241], and 5.22 [p. 245]; see also Figure 5.7 [p. 221])

Twelve pairs of cranial nerves emerge from the brain, passing through different cranial foramina to innervate structures of the head and neck. Some of these nerves, like the vagus, also innervate structures other than the head and neck, such as the thoracic and abdominal cavities.

Cranial nerves are numbered using Roman numerals from I to XII according to their location, from rostral to caudal:

I	Olfactory
II	Optic
III	Oculomotor
IV	Trochlear
V	Trigeminal
VI	Abducens
VII	Facial
VIII	Vestibulocochlear
IX	Glossopharyngeal
X	Vagus
XI	Accessory
XII	Hypoglossal

These nerves arise from the telencephalon (I), diencephalon (II), midbrain (III, IV), pons (V), pontomedullary junction (VI-VIII), and the medulla (IX-XII). Five (III, IV, VI, XI, XII) have a purely motor function; three (I, II, VIII) have a purely sensory function; and four (V, VII, IX, X) have a mixed function, both motor and sensory.

The cell bodies of first-order sensory neurons of cranial nerves (with the exception of nerves I and II) are collected in ganglia (e.g., trigeminal ganglion), and they synapse on second-order neurons within their respective brainstem cranial nerve nuclei. They next synapse on third-order sensory neurons in the thalamus. The cell bodies of the sensory neurons of cranial nerves I and II are located inside the organs that they innervate (nose and eyes).

With the exception of postganglionic visceral motor (parasympathetic) neurons, the cell bodies of all cranial nerve motor neurons are located in brainstem nuclei. Cranial nerve (and spinal nerve) motoneurons, in addition to their axons and the muscle fibers they innervate, form important functional units called *motor units*. Motor units represent the "final common pathway" for the control of movement (as termed by Charles Sherrington, a pioneering neurophysiologist).

Cranial Nerve Nuclei in Brainstem

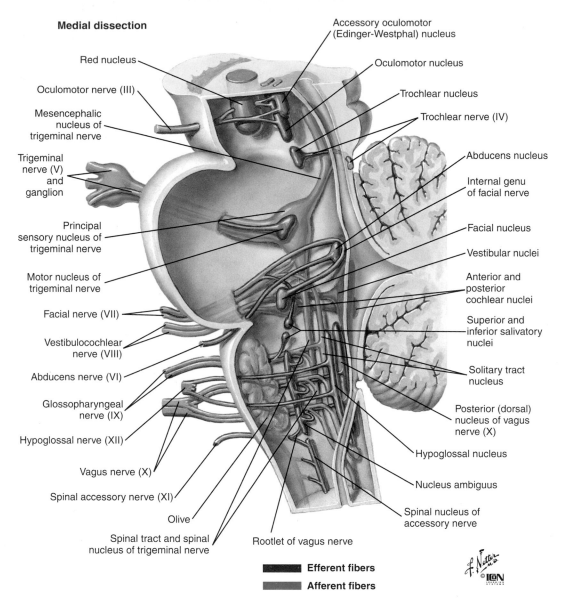

Medial dissection

Red nucleus

Oculomotor nerve (III)

Mesencephalic nucleus of trigeminal nerve

Trigeminal nerve (V) and ganglion

Principal sensory nucleus of trigeminal nerve

Motor nucleus of trigeminal nerve

Facial nerve (VII)

Vestibulocochlear nerve (VIII)

Abducens nerve (VI)

Glossopharyngeal nerve (IX)

Hypoglossal nerve (XII)

Vagus nerve (X)

Spinal accessory nerve (XI)

Olive

Spinal tract and spinal nucleus of trigeminal nerve

Accessory oculomotor (Edinger-Westphal) nucleus

Oculomotor nucleus

Trochlear nucleus

Trochlear nerve (IV)

Abducens nucleus

Internal genu of facial nerve

Facial nucleus

Vestibular nuclei

Anterior and posterior cochlear nuclei

Superior and inferior salivatory nuclei

Solitary tract nucleus

Posterior (dorsal) nucleus of vagus nerve (X)

Hypoglossal nucleus

Nucleus ambiguus

Spinal nucleus of accessory nerve

Rootlet of vagus nerve

███ **Efferent fibers**

███ **Afferent fibers**

Figure 5.19 Medial dissection of the brainstem cranial nerve nuclei and their efferent *(red)* and afferent *(blue)* fiber tracts.

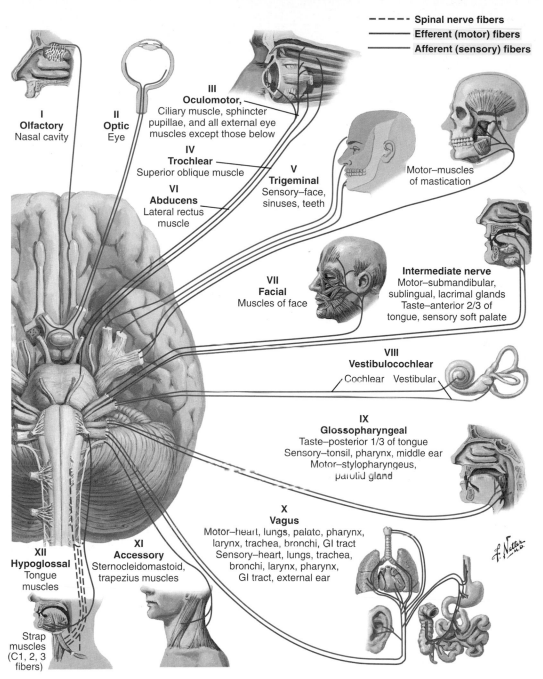

Figure 5.20. Motor and sensory distribution of the cranial nerves.

I Olfactory (Sensory)

The first-order olfactory neurons transmit signals from receptors in the region of the nasal mucosa through the cribriform plate of the ethmoid bone to synapse on second-order neurons in the olfactory bulb. Second-order olfactory fibers travel caudally through the olfactory tract, which runs underneath the frontal lobe; pass into the cerebral hemispheres; and terminate in the primary olfactory area, in the medial temporal lobe.

First-order neurons enter the cranial cavity through the cribriform plate of the ethmoid bone, and second-order neurons project to the cerebral cortex (telencephalon) through the olfactory tract. Function is special sensory: olfaction.

II Optic (Sensory)

The optic nerve originates from the retina. Its fibers course within the optic canal, which is formed by the posterior portion of the sphenoid bone, and converge to form the optic chiasm. The fibers then diverge into the optic tracts, which course toward the thalamus, where the fibers synapse in the lateral geniculate nucleus. The nerve fibers leave the thalamus to travel to the primary visual area in the occipital cortex.

The optic nerve enters the cranial cavity through the optic canal and enters the brain at the thalamus (diencephalon). Function is special sensory: vision.

III Oculomotor (Motor)

The oculomotor nerve emerges from the anterior mesencephalon (midbrain) and exits the cranial cavity through the superior orbital fissure of the sphenoid bone to enter into the orbit.

Function is as follows:
- Somatic motor: From the oculomotor nucleus located in the midbrain to the six extraocular eye muscles and the levator muscle of the upper eyelid
- Visceral motor: From the accessory oculomotor (Edinger-Westphal) nucleus located in the midbrain to the sphincter pupillae and ciliary muscles that are involved in the pupillary light and accommodation reflexes

IV Trochlear (Motor)

The smallest cranial nerve originates from the trochlear nucleus located in the midbrain and emerges from the posterior mesencephalon at the level of the inferior colliculus. Its fibers circle around the brainstem and course forward toward the eye in the subarachnoid space. Cranial nerve IV exits the cranial cavity and enters the orbit through the superior orbital fissure. The function of this nerve is somatic motor to the superior oblique muscle in the orbit.

V Trigeminal (Motor and Sensory) (Figures 5.21 [p. 244] and 5.22 [p. 245])

The trigeminal nerve is composed of three main divisions: ophthalmic, maxillary, and mandibular. These divisions converge at the level of the petrous portion of the temporal bone to form the trigeminal (or semilunar) ganglion. From the ganglion, the sensory fibers of the trigeminal nerve enter the brain at the metencephalon (pons) and terminate in the trigeminal sensory nucleus. The trigeminal sensory nucleus extends from the midbrain to the cervical spinal cord and is composed of three divisions: the mesencephalic nucleus, the principal sensory nucleus (located in the pons), and the spinal nucleus (located along the medulla and the upper portion of the cervical spinal cord). The motor component of the trigeminal originates from the motor nucleus of the trigeminal nerve located in the pons.

Special motor fibers (autonomic) from the facial and glossopharyngeal nerves terminate in ganglia (e.g., otic ganglion, submandibular ganglion, and pterygopalatine ganglion). The fibers originating from these ganglia that innervate the parotid, lacrimal, submandibular, and sublingual glands are part of the trigeminal nerve.

Ophthalmic Nerve, or Division (V1) (Sensory)

The cranial entry point of the ophthalmic nerve is the superior orbital fissure of the sphenoid bone.

The function is general sensory from the following areas: skin of the forehead, upper eyelid, and nose; mucous membranes of the anterior and superior portions of the nasal cavity and paranasal sinuses; and cornea of the eye.

Maxillary Nerve, or Division (V₂) (Sensory)

The cranial entry point of the maxillary nerve is the foramen rotundum of the sphenoid bone. The function is general sensory from the following areas: skin of the side of the forehead, the anterior cheek and the side of the nose, lower eyelid, upper lip, upper teeth, maxilla, palate, nasal septum, posterior and inferior portions of the nasal cavity, maxillary sinus, and gums and mucous membranes of the upper oral cavity.

Mandibular Nerve, or Division (V₃) (Sensory and Motor)

The cranial entry and exit point of the mandibular nerve is the foramen ovale of the sphenoid bone.

Its function is as follows:

- General sensory: From the anterior two-thirds of the tongue, mucous membranes of the floor of the mouth and the cheek, the lower teeth, part of the external ear (anterior part of the auricle, external acoustic meatus, external surface of the tympanic membrane), skin of the lower lip, the chin, the cheek, and the temple
- Branchial motor: To the muscles of mastication (masseter, temporalis, medial and lateral pterygoid), the mylohyoid, the anterior belly of the digastric, the tensor tympani, and the tensor veli palatini

Mesencephalic Trigeminal Pathway

Primary sensory neurons carry proprioceptive sensory information from the masticatory muscles and project primarily to the trigeminal motor nucleus for reflex control of masticatory movements.

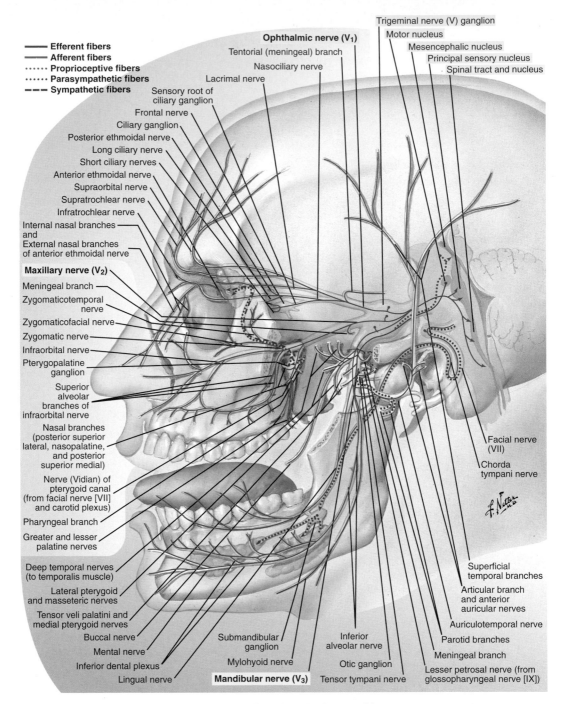

Figure 5.21. The trigeminal nerve (V).

— Efferent fibers
— Afferent fibers
••••• Proprioceptive fibers
••••• Parasympathetic fibers
– – – Sympathetic fibers

Ophthalmic nerve (V₁)
Tentorial (meningeal) branch
Nasociliary nerve
Lacrimal nerve
Sensory root of ciliary ganglion
Frontal nerve
Ciliary ganglion
Posterior ethmoidal nerve
Long ciliary nerve
Short ciliary nerves
Anterior ethmoidal nerve
Supraorbital nerve
Supratrochlear nerve
Infratrochlear nerve
Internal nasal branches and
External nasal branches of anterior ethmoidal nerve

Maxillary nerve (V₂)
Meningeal branch
Zygomaticotemporal nerve
Zygomaticofacial nerve
Zygomatic nerve
Infraorbital nerve
Pterygopalatine ganglion
Superior alveolar branches of infraorbital nerve
Nasal branches (posterior superior lateral, nasopalatine, and posterior superior medial)
Nerve (Vidian) of pterygoid canal (from facial nerve [VII] and carotid plexus)
Pharyngeal branch
Greater and lesser palatine nerves

Deep temporal nerves (to temporalis muscle)
Lateral pterygoid and masseteric nerves
Tensor veli palatini and medial pterygoid nerves
Buccal nerve
Mental nerve
Inferior dental plexus
Lingual nerve

Trigeminal nerve (V) ganglion
Motor nucleus
Mesencephalic nucleus
Principal sensory nucleus
Spinal tract and nucleus

Facial nerve (VII)
Chorda tympani nerve

Superficial temporal branches
Articular branch and anterior auricular nerves
Auriculotemporal nerve
Parotid branches
Meningeal branch
Lesser petrosal nerve (from glossopharyngeal nerve [IX])

Submandibular ganglion
Mylohyoid nerve
Mandibular nerve (V₃)
Inferior alveolar nerve
Otic ganglion
Tensor tympani nerve

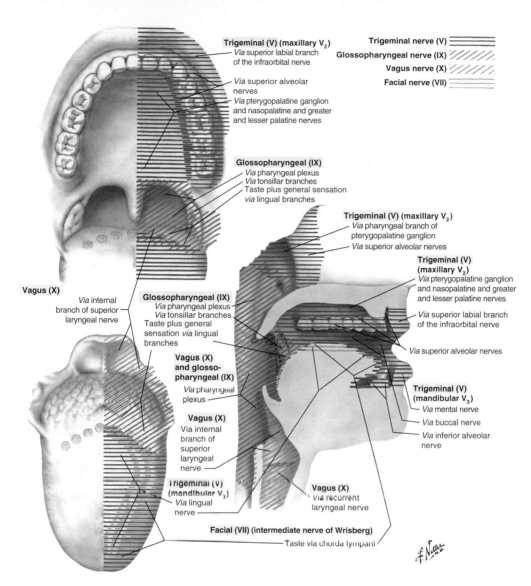

Figure 5.22. Sensory innervation of the oral cavity, larynx and pharynx.

VI Abducens (Motor)

The abducens nerve, which originates from the abducens nucleus (located in the pons), emerges from the inferior part of the pons and enters the orbit to reach the eye. The brain exit point is the junction between the metencephalon (pons) and the myelencephalon (medulla), and the cranial exit point is the superior orbital fissure of the sphenoid bone.

Function is somatic motor: To the lateral rectus muscle of the ipsilateral orbit.

VII Facial (Motor and Sensory) (Figure 5.23; see also Figure 5.22 [p. 245])

The facial nerve travels from the pons to enter the temporal bone and emerges from the cranium as five distinct branches. The brain exit point is the junction between the metencephalon (pons) and the myelencephalon (medulla). For the cranial exit point, the nerve runs in the internal acoustic meatus and the facial canal in the petrous part of the temporal bone and leaves the skull through the stylomastoid foramen.

Function is mixed, as follows:
- General sensory: From the skin of the concha of the auricle and external acoustic meatus to the spinal nucleus of the trigeminal nerve
- Special sensory: Taste information from the anterior two-thirds of the tongue to the solitary tract nucleus located in the medulla
- Branchial motor: From the motor nucleus of the facial nerve (located in the pons) to the muscles of facial expression (excluding the primary muscles of mastication), the stylohyoid, the posterior belly of the digastric, and the stapedius muscle
- Visceral motor: From the superior salivatory nucleus (located in the pons) as preganglionic autonomic fibers to the mucous membranes of the hard and soft palate and nose, in addition to the lacrimal, submandibular, and sublingual glands

Several terminal branches of the facial nerves join to form the parotid plexus, which is located in the parotid salivary gland. The nerve passes into the gland and divides into several branches: temporal, zygomatic, buccal, mandibular, and cervical.

The motor nucleus of the facial nerve can be divided in two portions. The upper portion (which innervates muscles in the upper part of the face) receives innervation from both cerebral hemispheres. In contrast, the lower portion of the nucleus (which innervates muscles in the lower part of the face) receives mainly contralateral cortical innervation.

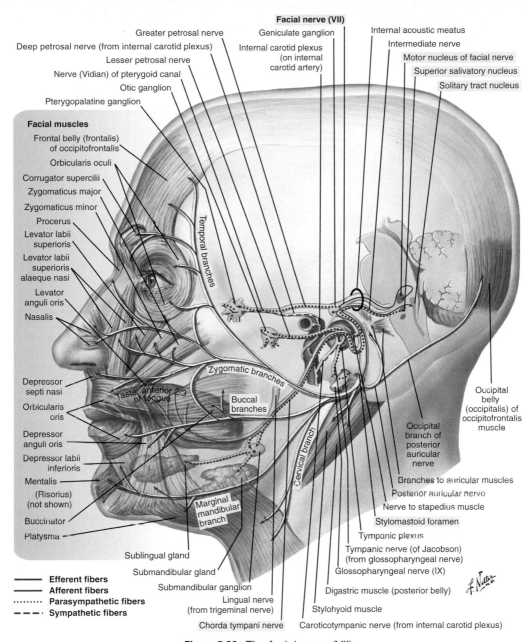

Figure 5.23. The facial nerve (VII).

VIII Vestibulocochlear (Sensory) (Figure 5.24)

The vestibulocochlear nerve originates from the internal ear, located in the temporal bone, runs through the internal acoustic meatus, enters in the brainstem at the level of the junction between the metencephalon (pons) and the myelencephalon (medulla), and terminates in the vestibular nuclei and cochlear nuclei (located in the pontomedullary junction). The nerve fibers originating from the auditory receptors in the cochlea form the cochlear nerve, and the nerve fibers originating from the equilibrium receptors in the semicircular canals and vestibule form the vestibular nerve. These two nerves fuse to form the vestibulocochlear nerve. The cranial entry point is the internal acoustic meatus, and the brain entry point is the junction between the metencephalon (pons) and the myelencephalon (medulla).

Function is special sensory for audition, balance, and body orientation.

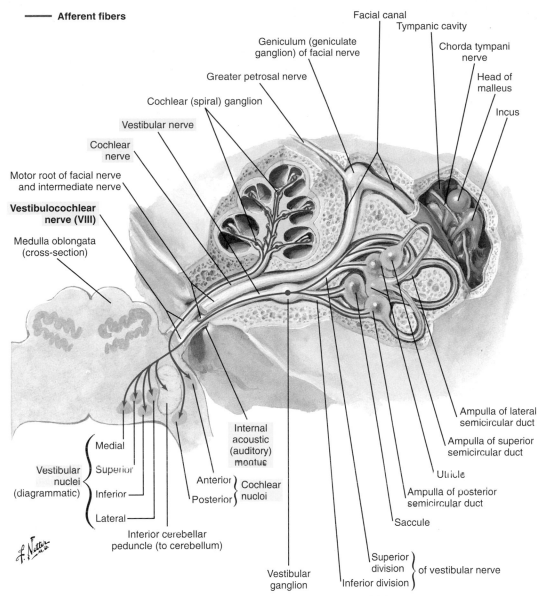

Afferent fibers

Facial canal
Tympanic cavity
Geniculum (geniculate ganglion) of facial nerve
Chorda tympani nerve
Greater petrosal nerve
Head of malleus
Cochlear (spiral) ganglion
Incus
Vestibular nerve
Cochlear nerve
Motor root of facial nerve and intermediate nerve
Vestibulocochlear nerve (VIII)
Medulla oblongata (cross-section)

Ampulla of lateral semicircular duct
Ampulla of superior semicircular duct
Internal acoustic (auditory) meatus
Utricle
Ampulla of posterior semicircular duct

Medial
Vestibular nuclei (diagrammatic)
Superior
Anterior
Cochlear nucloi
Inferior
Posterior
Saccule
Lateral
Interior cerebellar peduncle (to cerebellum)
Superior division
of vestibular nerve
Vestibular ganglion
Inferior division

Figure 5.24. The vestibulocochlear nerve (VIII).

IX Glossopharyngeal (Motor and Sensory) (Figure 5.25; see also Figure 5.22 [p. 245])

The glossopharyngeal nerve emerges from the myelencephalon (medulla) and courses from the cranium to the pharynx. The brain exit point of cranial nerve IX is the myelencephalon (medulla), and the cranial exit point is the jugular foramen, between the temporal bone and the occipital bone.

Function is mixed, as follows:

- Branchial motor: From the nucleus ambiguus (located in the medulla) to the stylopharyngeus muscle
- Visceral motor: From the inferior salivatory nucleus (located in the medulla) as preganglionic autonomic fibers to the parotid gland
- General sensory: From the posterior one-third of the tongue, the tonsils, the pharynx, the tympanic membrane (internal surface), the tympanic cavity, and the pharyngotympanic tube to the spinal nucleus of the trigeminal nerve
- Visceral sensory: From the carotid body and sinus to the solitary tract nucleus
- Special sensory: Taste from the posterior one-third of the tongue to the solitary tract nucleus

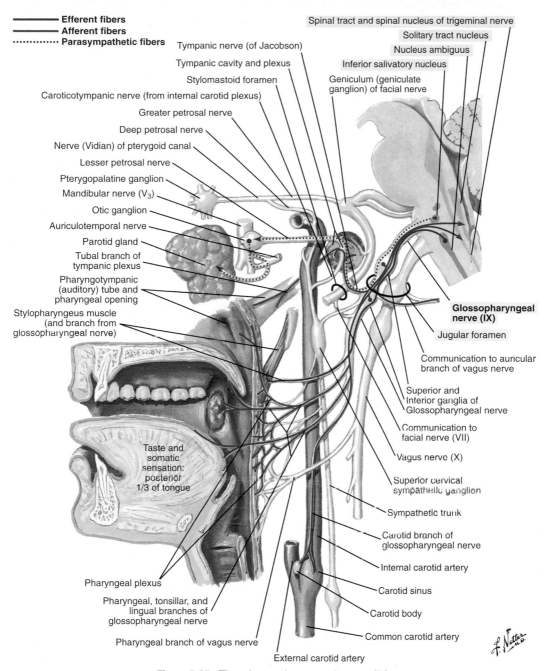

Figure 5.25. The glossopharyngeal nerve (IX).

X Vagus, or Pneumogastric, Nerve (Motor and Sensory) (Figure 5.26; see also Figure 5.22 [p. 245])

The vagus nerve emerges from the medulla; travels down to the jugular foramen; and continues its course down to the neck, thorax, and abdomen. The brain exit point is the myelencephalon (medulla), and the cranial exit point is the jugular foramen, between the temporal bone and the occipital bone.

Function is mixed, as follows:

- Branchial motor: From the nucleus ambiguus to the muscles of the pharynx (except the stylopharyngeus, which is innervated by the glossopharyngeal nerve), muscles of the larynx, and muscles of the soft palate (except the tensor veli palatini, which is innervated by the trigeminal nerve)
- Visceral motor: From the posterior (dorsal) nucleus (located in the medulla) to smooth muscle and glands of the pharynx, larynx, and viscera of the thorax and abdomen, including smooth muscle of the esophagus and cardiac muscle
- General sensory: From portions of the skin of the external ear and external acoustic meatus, part of the external surface of the tympanic membrane, pharynx and larynx, and dura mater of the posterior cranial fossa to terminate in the spinal nucleus of the trigeminal nerve
- Visceral sensory: From the larynx (above and below the vocal folds), esophagus, trachea, heart, and thoracic and abdominal viscera (including the lungs and gastrointestinal tract) to the solitary tract nucleus
- Special sensory: Taste information from the epiglottis and pharynx to the solitary tract nucleus

Vagus Nerve (X)

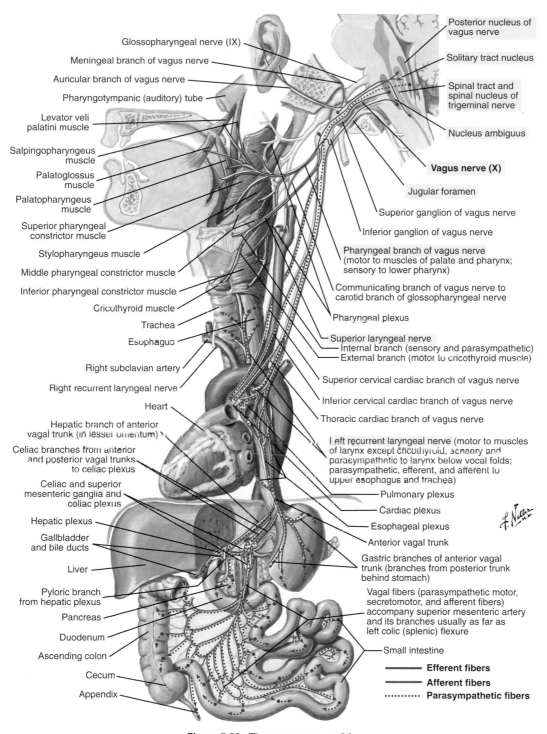

Glossopharyngeal nerve (IX)

Meningeal branch of vagus nerve

Auricular branch of vagus nerve

Pharyngotympanic (auditory) tube

Levator veli palatini muscle

Salpingopharyngeus muscle

Palatoglossus muscle

Palatopharyngeus muscle

Superior pharyngeal constrictor muscle

Stylopharyngeus muscle

Middle pharyngeal constrictor muscle

Inferior pharyngeal constrictor muscle

Cricothyroid muscle

Trachea

Esophagus

Right subclavian artery

Right recurrent laryngeal nerve

Heart

Hepatic branch of anterior vagal trunk (in lesser omentum)

Celiac branches from anterior and posterior vagal trunks to celiac plexus

Celiac and superior mesenteric ganglia and celiac plexus

Hepatic plexus

Gallbladder and bile ducts

Liver

Pyloric branch from hepatic plexus

Pancreas

Duodenum

Ascending colon

Cecum

Appendix

Posterior nucleus of vagus nerve

Solitary tract nucleus

Spinal tract and spinal nucleus of trigeminal nerve

Nucleus ambiguus

Vagus nerve (X)

Jugular foramen

Superior ganglion of vagus nerve

Inferior ganglion of vagus nerve

Pharyngeal branch of vagus nerve (motor to muscles of palate and pharynx; sensory to lower pharynx)

Communicating branch of vagus nerve to carotid branch of glossopharyngeal nerve

Pharyngeal plexus

Superior laryngeal nerve
Internal branch (sensory and parasympathetic)
External branch (motor to cricothyroid muscle)

Superior cervical cardiac branch of vagus nerve

Inferior cervical cardiac branch of vagus nerve

Thoracic cardiac branch of vagus nerve

Left recurrent laryngeal nerve (motor to muscles of larynx except cricothyroid, sensory and parasympathetic to larynx below vocal folds; parasympathetic, efferent, and afferent to upper esophagus and trachea)

Pulmonary plexus

Cardiac plexus

Esophageal plexus

Anterior vagal trunk

Gastric branches of anterior vagal trunk (branches from posterior trunk behind stomach)

Vagal fibers (parasympathetic motor, secretomotor, and afferent fibers) accompany superior mesenteric artery and its branches usually as far as left colic (splenic) flexure

Small intestine

━━━━ **Efferent fibers**
━━━━ **Afferent fibers**
·········· **Parasympathetic fibers**

Figure 5.26. The vagus nerve (X).

XI Spinal Accessory (Motor) (Figure 5.27)

The spinal accessory nerve arises from the upper five or six cervical segments of the spinal cord (spinal nucleus of the accessory nerve) and enters the skull through the foramen magnum. The nerve exits through the jugular foramen, between the temporal bone and the occipital bone.

Function is branchial motor: To the trapezius and sternocleidomastoid muscles.

Spinal Accessory Nerve (XI)

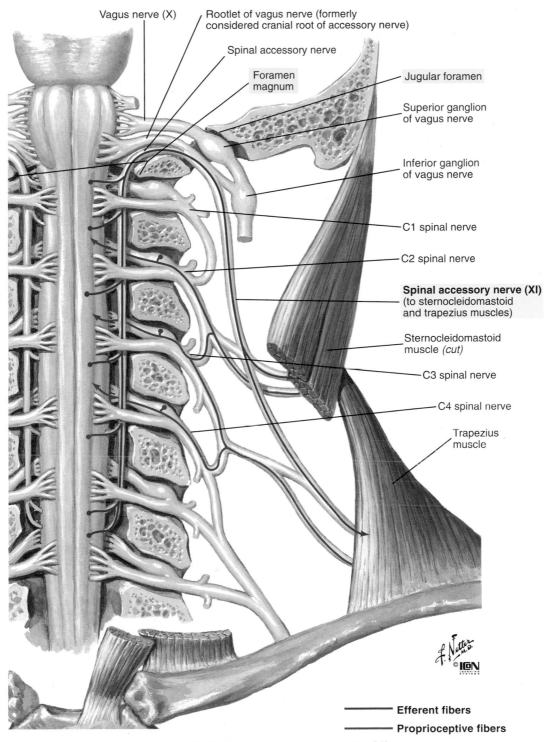

Vagus nerve (X)

Rootlet of vagus nerve (formerly considered cranial root of accessory nerve)

Spinal accessory nerve

Foramen magnum

Jugular foramen

Superior ganglion of vagus nerve

Inferior ganglion of vagus nerve

C1 spinal nerve

C2 spinal nerve

Spinal accessory nerve (XI) (to sternocleidomastoid and trapezius muscles)

Sternocleidomastoid muscle *(cut)*

C3 spinal nerve

C4 spinal nerve

Trapezius muscle

———— Efferent fibers

———— Proprioceptive fibers

Figure 5.27. The spinal accessory nerve (XI).

XII Hypoglossal (Motor) (Figure 5.28)

The hypoglossal nerve originates from the hypoglossal nucleus located in the medulla and innervates muscles of the tongue. The brain exit point of the hypoglossal is the myelencephalon (medulla), and the cranial exit point is the hypoglossal canal in the occipital bone.

Function is branchial motor: To all intrinsic muscles of the tongue and three of the four extrinsic muscles of the tongue—genioglossus, hyoglossus, and styloglossus. The fourth muscle, the palatoglossus, is supplied by the vagus nerve.

The omohyoid, sternohyoid, and sternothyroid muscles are innervated by cervical nerves C1-C3 (via the ansa hypoglossi or ansa cervicalis). The geniohyoid and thyrohyoid muscles are innervated by C1 nerves, not via the ansa cervicalis. The nerve fibers to these muscles can be found coursing with the hypoglossal nerve.

Although the nucleus of the hypoglossal nerve receives predominantly contralateral cortical innervation, the medial part of the nucleus (innervating the genioglossus and the transverse and vertical intrinsic tongue muscles) receives bilateral innervation.

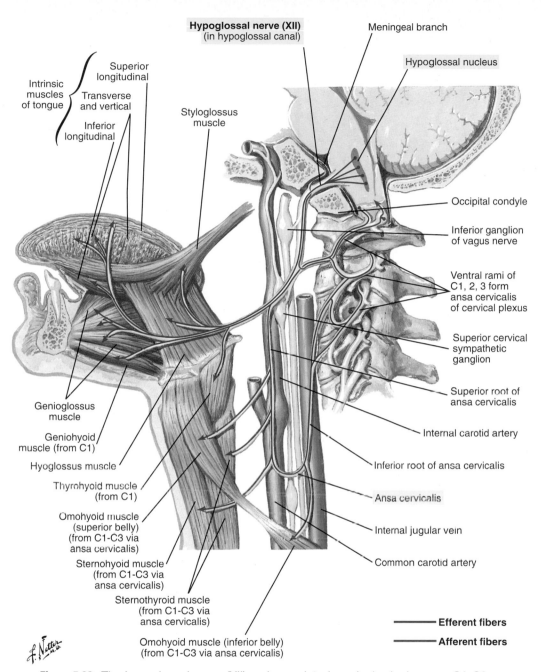

Hypoglossal nerve (XII)
(in hypoglossal canal)

Meningeal branch

Hypoglossal nucleus

Intrinsic
muscles
of tongue

Superior
longitudinal

Transverse
and vertical

Inferior
longitudinal

Styloglossus
muscle

Occipital condyle

Inferior ganglion
of vagus nerve

Ventral rami of
C1, 2, 3 form
ansa cervicalis
of cervical plexus

Superior cervical
sympathetic
ganglion

Superior root of
ansa cervicalis

Internal carotid artery

Inferior root of ansa cervicalis

Genioglossus
muscle

Geniohyoid
muscle (from C1)

Hyoglossus muscle

Thyrohyoid muscle
(from C1)

Omohyoid muscle
(superior belly)
(from C1-C3 via
ansa cervicalis)

Sternohyoid muscle
(from C1-C3 via
ansa cervicalis)

Sternothyroid muscle
(from C1-C3 via
ansa cervicalis)

Omohyoid muscle (inferior belly)
(from C1-C3 via ansa cervicalis)

Ansa cervicalis

Internal jugular vein

Common carotid artery

——— **Efferent fibers**
——— **Afferent fibers**

Figure 5.28. The hypoglossal nerve (XII) and associated cervical spinal nerves C1-C3.

■ SPINAL NERVES

Thirty-one pairs of spinal nerves emerge from the spinal cord to innervate the structures of the trunk (including the muscles of respiration) and the lower and upper limbs:

- C1-C8 (8 cervical)
- T1-T12 (12 thoracic)
- L1-L5 (5 lumbar)
- S1-S5 (5 sacral)
- Co (1 coccygeal)

The motor and sensory fibers of the spinal nerves emerge, respectively, from the ventral and dorsal horns of the spinal cord as nerve rootlets, which converge to form two roots: a ventral root and a dorsal root. These two roots merge as they exit the vertebral canal, then divide again into two rami: a ventral ramus and a dorsal ramus. Globally, the ventral rami innervate the lower and upper limbs, in addition to the muscles and skin of the anterior part of the trunk. The dorsal rami innervate the muscles and skin of the back.

Cell bodies of motor fibers are located in the ventral horns (gray matter) of the spinal cord (see Figure 5.8 [p. 223]). Cell bodies of sensory fibers are located in dorsal root ganglia.

Summary of Cranial Nerves Significant to Speech, Mastication/Swallowing, and Hearing

Cranial Nerves	Functions and Structures Supplied	Nuclei Location
V Trigeminal (sensory/motor) (see Figures 5.21 [p. 244] and 5.22 [p. 245]) Three divisions: 1. Ophthalmic 2. Maxillary 3. Mandibular	*Sensory:* face, mouth, palate, teeth, nasal cavity, and anterior two-thirds of the tongue *Motor:* muscles of mastication (except the posterior belly of the digastric and geniohyoid), the mylohyoid, the tensor veli palatini, and the tensor tympani	*Sensory:* extends from the midbrain to the spinal cord *Motor:* in the pons
VII Facial (sensory/motor) (see Figures 5.22 [p. 245] and 5.23 [p. 247])	*Sensory:* skin of the concha of the auricle and external acoustic meatus *Motor:* muscles of facial expression and nasal muscles, posterior belly of the digastric, stylohyoid, and stapedius muscle; responsible for facial muscle tone *Secretory:* for the lacrimal, submandibular, and sublingual glands and mucous membranes for palate and nose *Taste:* from anterior two-thirds of the tongue	*Sensory:* extends from the midbrain to the spinal cord *Motor and Secretory:* in the pons *Taste:* in the medulla
VIII Vestibulocochlear (sensory) (see Figure 5.24 [p. 249])	*Sensory:* from auditory (cochlear branch) and equilibrium (vestibular branch) receptors	*Sensory:* at the pontomedullary junction
IX Glossopharyngeal (sensory/motor) (see Figures 5.22 [p. 245] and 5.25 [p. 251])	*Sensory:* from the posterior one-third of the tongue, pharynx, tonsils, internal surface of tympanic membrane, tympanic cavity, pharyngotympanic tube *Motor:* to the stylopharyngeus muscle *Secretory:* for the parotid gland *Taste:* from the posterior one-third of the tongue	*Sensory:* extends from the midbrain to the spinal cord *Motor, Secretory, and Taste:* in the medulla
X Vagus (sensory/motor) (see Figures 5.22 [p. 245] and 5.26 [p. 253])	*Sensory:* from larynx and pharynx, thorax, abdomen, external surface of tympanic membrane, part of external ear and external acoustic meatus *Motor:* to intrinsic laryngeal, pharyngeal (except stylopharyngeus), soft palate (except tensor veli palatini), and esophageal muscles *Taste:* from the epiglottic region and the root of the tongue	*Sensory:* extends from the midbrain to the spinal cord *Motor and Taste:* in the medulla
XI Spinal accessory (motor) (see Figure 5.27 [p. 255])	*Motor:* to trapezius and sternocleidomastoid	*Motor:* from the upper five or six cervical segments of the spinal cord
XII Hypoglossal (motor) (see Figure 5.28 [p. 257])	*Motor:* to all intrinsic and most extrinsic muscles of the tongue (except the palatoglossus)	*Motor:* in the medulla

INDEX

Note: Page numbers followed by '*f*' indicate figures those followed by '*t*' indicate tables.